dementia is different

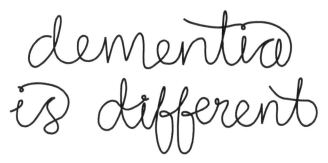

dementia is different

Not just another ordinary illness

Ludomyr Mykyta

AUSTRALIAN SCHOLARLY

First published 2018 by
Australian Scholarly Publishing Pty Ltd

7 Lt Lothian St Nth, North Melbourne, Vic 3051

Tel: 03 9329 6963 / Fax: 03 9329 5452
enquiry@scholarly.info / www.scholarly.info

ISBN 978-1-925801-24-8

Cover design: Sarah Anderson

Contents

Foreword

Confused about dementia?

Dr Lu Mykyta's extensive experience and razor sharp intellect provide answers in plain language to the many questions causing concern about this growing epidemic.

Experiencing problems navigating the aged care system?

This book is for you. Whether you are an aged care professional or a carer providing help to those in need, there are multiple examples from real life situations of successful interventions in problems experienced by patients, clients and providers.

Are you a research worker or policy provider to government in the areas of dementia, diabetes mellitus or another chronic illness?

Dr Mykyta's involvement in policy and operations in the World Health Organisation, and in the Commonwealth and State governments in Australia, equips him to raise pertinent questions and provide ideas and options to improve health care in Australia at this challenging time.

After a career in the military and the public service, I had the great good fortune to work for Dr Mykyta when he was the Director of the South Australian Western Domiciliary Care Service.

If only this book had been available to me then!

Dr Keith Fleming

Preface

This book was born in a fit of rage. During a busy rural visit, I became outraged by the cruel and callous way that one particular old lady had been treated by her general practitioner. She had been reluctant to see anybody, and he had then threatened her, telling her that she had Alzheimer's disease, and if she did not do as he said, he would put her in a nursing home. Her family confirmed that that was how the appointment had been set up. She was petrified and needed a lot of comforting before we could proceed. Fear of placement is more than common amongst the patients that I see.

In this day and age, fear of placement is not, nor should it be, the probable outcome of the consultation for most of the people that we see. After the visit and stopping to think (advice that I am always giving harassed partners and relatives), I realised that what had so enraged me had been a symptom, or sign, of a much deeper malaise that I perceive in the healthcare system.

For a long time, I have harboured misgivings about the way that patients with dementia were being managed in general, not just in this one. Over the years, I have been referred many patients seen by other mainstream practitioners in the field, including neurologists, psycho-geriatricians and, alas, even other geriatricians, who had been tagged with clever labels, but whose presenting concerns had not been fully elucidated, addressed, explained, or resolved. I doubt that they had even been understood.

A close friend and colleague who read and gave me feedback about previous versions of the document had asked me what I was trying to do, write a scientific treatise or a biography? Who was my audience?

Such a pivotal question deserves answers. At first it was simply, 'all of the above'. I finally decided that what I was describing was my evolution into the geriatrician that I wished to become. There is no end, because I am still evolving and will continue to evolve until the day I finally retire. Learning from experience fuels this evolution, and I am fully persuaded by the adage, 'living is learning'.

Who is my audience? For many years throughout my clinical career I was a very active member of the Australian Association of Gerontology and the International Association of Gerontology, and I was the program director of a World Congress of Gerontology. Through gerontology I greatly extended my range of knowledge and interest and I had the opportunity to interact with many different academic and care professionals. Hence an obvious part of my target audience is the sort of people who come to a Gerontology conference, namely those interested in gerontology from every perspective.

I also spend a lot of time and effort explaining what is happening to patients, partners, relatives, and carers. At the conclusion of my assessments, they know exactly what will be in the report that I will send to their general practitioner. I therefore include them in my target audience.

More succinctly, I am aiming at anyone who participates in dementia care at any level, or has to live with its consequences. I have worked hard to make myself comprehensible to patients and life partners, and I hope that I will not be writing anything too esoteric for most intelligent people to understand.

In my more than fifty years of practice, I have met and got to know literally thousands of patients, partners, relatives, and carers and have addressed and participated in numerous Carer Groups. Many of the partners and carers who I met and continue to meet had been dissatisfied with the treatment that they had received from medical practitioners and health and aged care services. No doubt my age, and the looming end of my career, has also influenced my resolve to get many things off my chest before it is too late.

I did not set out to write a textbook. Indeed, I deliberately set out to write 'not a textbook'. This work reflects my views about the nature of Medicine in general, and Geriatric Medicine and how it should be practised in particular. It reflects the way that I reason and practice, and the way that I teach students and educate patients and relatives. I chose to focus on dementia because it is quintessentially a complex chronic condition that requires all the skills, attitudes and values that I believe a geriatrician must possess.

As a student, I used to frequent the Red Cross bookshop in Adelaide. The first reason had been to buy another yard of 'thruppenny' books (they had to be romantic novels written before the Great War) for the ancient landlady of a friend from medical school. That is how I discovered that the bookshop also had a lot of medical books, probably from deceased estates, and I bought a good many. One book, written by a paediatric cardiothoracic surgeon, had a lasting impact. I could not appreciate its technical merits, but it was extraordinarily readable, and I was struck by the sheer humanity of the author. I cannot remember his name but I do remember that even a super-specialist could be a dedicated and humanitarian doctor.

Textbooks are written to a formula that greatly narrows what can be written and pass the peer-review processes before it can be published. I wish to challenge the norms and standards that 'peers' will apply. I will even question the bona fides of these peers and point out the shortcomings of the opinions and beliefs that they represent.

Anyone expecting a standard textbook will therefore be disappointed that I do not go into details of demographic trends, that I make only passing reference to the various forms of dementia, and that there is minimal discussion of imaging and investigation. These are deliberate omissions. I wish to demonstrate that the conventional way of managing dementia as described in mainstream text books is fundamentally flawed, and that rather than being totally dependent on the conventional version of the science of medicine, we should learn how to use the art more effectively.

I also did not want to write a textbook because I did not want to feel obliged to reference every statement or opinion, although some references are inevitable. This is not entirely because I am too lazy to do all the unavoidable searching (I have done a huge amount of study), but because there is now a belief within the professions that requires every concept, idea, observation, intervention, et cetera, to have been 'proved' before it has any legitimacy. I want the readers to decide what is believable, and what is consistent with their values, intuitive beliefs, and world views. Requiring 'proof' from references restricts free thinking to what is allowable, namely current dogma.

Since this is not a textbook, I will continue to make my disclaimers now, rather than at the end of the book. I have always been passionate about my work. As a student, I was an unashamed idealist. I tackled issues of social justice at every opportunity. For me it was all very clear. It was black or it was white, and there were no shades of grey. I later recalled heated debates with my father with shame for not understanding that he too had been an idealist, who had paid much more dearly for his beliefs than I ever could, but had learnt to temper his utterances with understanding, tolerance of others, and reason.

Very early in my career, during my internship, I was labelled an angry young man, because I regularly openly challenged a particular clinical and academic senior on ward rounds and other clinical gatherings because I objected to the way that he treated our patients. He was focused on his research projects and virtually ignored patients who did not suit his current agenda. I did not respect him, and I could not think of him as a mentor or a role model. The senior registrar who held the unit together more closely fitted that role.

Throughout my career I have challenged authority, bureaucracy, and my political masters. I gradually evolved from that angry young man until I achieved my current designation of 'grumpy old man'. As time went by, my growing seniority made me a truly irritating nuisance who could not be readily dismissed, irrespective of what my place was within the system.

Grumpy is better than angry, because it implies less impulsiveness and more controlled passion, but no loss of the driving idealism; and the term is often meant to be affectionate. Old can mean 'elder', someone whose opinions may be worth listening to, but who can be ignored if preferred without career consequences. Grumpy old people can dare and afford to be iconoclasts.

On a more serious note, the most precious asset that we old codgers have is what I call a corporate memory. We have been around for a long time and we have seen and experienced many things, good, bad, and indifferent. We have a history, a longitudinal perspective that for me extends over half a century. Like my contemporaries, I have seen our health system evolve. It is said that there is no such thing as a new joke. Much the same can be said about modern healthcare reform.

In recent times, for largely political reasons, any 'reform' that is introduced must be seen to be new and innovative: to maximise photo opportunities and kudos for the Minister. This leads to a sort of cognitive neglect of history. When I have taught health planning I always said that the first step was: Do your homework. Find out how this issue is being dealt with now, and by whom. I could cite many examples where something that had been done very well and very effectively in the past has been completely ignored in the name of innovation.

Finding fault with conventional wisdom and practice requires us to challenge the authority that educates and administers our profession, and there is nothing as conventional and conservative as that authority. This is inevitable because it is self-perpetuating. Like is replaced with like when a vacancy arises. It has few attributes that allow the merest intimation that it could just possibly be in error.

As a profession, we are and always have been conventional and compliant with current orthodoxy and dogma. Being a surviving iconoclast involves good timing. Grumpy old men and women are not looking for career opportunity, tenure and promotion, and they are secure enough in their self-worth and self-esteem not to care too much about what others may think of them.

I will now expand on my positive attributes. I avoid political correctness like the plague that it is, and I trust that the reader will not be mortally offended when I randomly use 'he' or 'she' instead of he/she, and talk about patients, not clients. By nature, I am not a racist, or a bigot, nor do I discriminate against any minority. I do have dislikes. A short list contains racists, bigots, those who discriminate against minorities, and zealots of all persuasions. Hmm, perhaps I do discriminate against some minorities. I also hate insensitivity, cruelty, callousness, and unfairness. I despise smugness and ignorance in those purporting to be wise. I pity people who are humourless and take themselves too seriously.

On another serious note, I must proclaim that I believe in the practice of not only evidence-based medicine, but evidence-based healthcare as a whole. I believe in the scientific method and only a fool would fail to recognise the dramatic achievements of researchers in every field of medicine, and dementia in particular. I do however have concerns about the narrow range of what we conventionally recognise and accept as representing legitimate science as applied to clinical practice.

I realise that I am challenging many entrenched beliefs, and that my manner may seem confronting to those I question and criticise. Anyone who reads this whole book should realise that I am not just iconoclastically tearing down idols, or venting my spleen, I am offering different ways of looking at and doing things. While it is human nature to react to criticism defensively and resentfully, I remind the reader that it takes a true scientist to accept the possibility that the critic may be right to some degree, and that there is at least a slight chance that we may be wrong. What the true scientist would do is analyse the criticism and try to learn from it.

One obvious question that arises is how can any new idea originate in our controlled and guideline-driven intellectual and practice environment? In the early literature on guideline development, the opinions of leaders in a given field were accepted as evidence even though there was little, if any, supporting research or literature available to cite.

I am regularly gratified to find that something that I have been doing intuitively for years has finally been researched, 'proved', and found its way into guidelines. I suspect that anyone who has been practising as long as I, regularly finds the same thing. This is not just an idle boast. My writings and teachings go back a long way and I could produce documented evidence that supports what I am claiming if challenged. It should however not be too surprising that something that makes intuitive sense to an experienced practitioner, is likely to occur to more than one at any given time.

I have had a very long career with no end in sight, although I always say that I plan to practice for a further five years in workforce surveys. I have been doing this for some time. I have no succession plan. I have been criticised for this. As a sole practitioner in private practice it is well-nigh impossible for me to have a succession plan. I believe that that is the responsibility of the healthcare system, and I will discuss this point in another chapter. The fact that there is no succession plan is probably the main reason that I put off retirement. No one who replaced me would hold the views that I hold so passionately as described in this book.

In the early years of my career I had the opportunity to dabble in several specialties including inter-alia: pathology, general medicine, cardiology, gastroenterology, intensive care, and even psychiatry. I trained and qualified in Internal Medicine, and sub-specialised in Geriatric Medicine and Rehabilitation Medicine.

As a clinician, senior medical administrator in various public services, and as a WHO consultant, I have had the unique opportunity to analyse health care systems, structures, health units, and the way that specific conditions were managed at the national, state, regional, local and personal level in several countries.

I have established or headed up services at national, state, regional and local level. At all times, I have been an active clinical participant. I did not expect others to do anything that I was not prepared to do myself. I venture to suggest that this is not the way that services are being established now. The medical profession is being distanced from the creation and management of the health system. I have had it seriously put to me by senior (lay) bureaucrats and politicians that 'Healthcare is too important to be left to doctors'. Obviously non-practising lawyers, accountants, and business entrepreneurs are more appropriate.

Because I come from a small city, in a small state (population-wise that is, in geographical area it is about 10% of the size of Europe), critics may argue that I am describing what happens in a backwater, and a small pond, and does not reflect what happens in their larger and more important centres.

Oceans are made of many small ponds, and as I don't tire of telling anyone who will listen, that it is easier to get job satisfaction working in rural towns, as I do, because of the tightness of communication, true teamwork, true community spirit, and distance from the mindless bureaucracy and fortified fiefdoms that I find in big cities. With the information revolution in full swing, limitations in the distribution of health services on the grounds of location and distance are becoming specious and irrelevant rationalisations. However, the ease with which clinical communication can be made electronically from afar is a growing threat to the practice of face-to-face medicine, which is ultimately the most fundamental element in clinical medicine. E-medicine is a tool of trade.

It is inevitable that a geriatrician would become interested in dementia. I am past the retirement age, and since my resignation from the Public Service some 12 years ago, I decided that I would more or less exclusively devote myself to the management of dementia in all settings. Prior to this, I had had a long experience in Psychogeriatrics, having been the visiting Geriatrician to state psychiatric hospitals and a multidisciplinary psychogeriatric unit and memory clinic in a private psychiatric hospital for many years. This unit also had a research arm, and we participated in several dementia-related multinational drug trials.

I have had a long experience in rural and remote South Australia. I have been visiting some country centres for well over 30 years and have a long service medal from the Rural Doctors Workforce Agency to prove it. In the metropolitan area, I now largely restrict myself to dealing with behavioural issues in residential facilities. In the course of my work I visit hospitals, residential facilities, and homes. I also see patients in clinics, community health centres and my rooms. I can honestly say that I have personally seen several thousand dementia sufferers and their families in all settings (I have close to 10,000 records created since I have been using electronic records).

In other incarnations, I have had a more than working knowledge of rural New South Wales, Queensland and the Northern Territory. In South Australia, rural and remote means just that. There are only three centres with populations over 20,000 outside the Adelaide metropolitan area. The furthest centre that I used to visit regularly had been 777 km away. I fly where I can, and drive where I can't. Only the largest centres are accessible by air, so I spend a lot of time in my car.

In the country, as in the city, there are many patients who refuse to see doctors in their usual workplaces. It becomes necessary to visit them in their settings and persuade them to agree to be seen – 'if the mountain won't come to Mohammad …' For this, and many other reasons that I will explain later, I believe that patients should be seen where they live or lie, particularly when questions are raised about their capacity to continue to manage safely in that situation.

I probably do more home visits than any modern general practitioner. For example, I have driven 60 km from a country town to a farmhouse along a dirt road, and interviewed an elderly man sitting on a crate in his shed. He offered me a beer and had three or four while we talked. I declined the offer. We had to talk in his shed because he refused to go into the house except to eat and sleep. He was angry with his daughter, who had given up her job in Adelaide and moved in to care for him after his wife died, because 'she is trying to run my life'. There were major concerns about his health, but he would not agree to be taken to the nearest town to see his local doctor. He continued to drive his ute to the nearest pub to stock up on beer. This necessitated crossing a major highway. On his arrival at the pub, he not only stocked up, but had a few beers as well. The publican could not be persuaded to sell him less beer at a sitting. He was at no risk of being seen in a multidisciplinary memory clinic where all the latest investigational and imaging modalities were available, and where cross-referrals for specialist opinions were routine. He eventually lost his driver's licence after being breathalysed on one of his trips to the pub.

I have visited an old man who lived in a car body in a paddock on a tolerant farmer's property. I have visited numerous old ladies who lived in appalling squalor, usually with a colony of feral cats.

The thing that all these people had in common was that they desperately needed to be seen by a doctor, and there was no way that they would present in rooms, community health centres, memory clinics, or any hospital. It could be argued that they are the people in the greatest need of our intervention, but least likely to receive it.

Many residents of aged care facilities are unfit to travel any distance. This is not just a rural phenomenon. Their chances of being seen and properly assessed by a visiting specialist are minimal at best, and the only contribution that some leading geriatricians and psychogeriatricians make is to criticize the quality of their care with vitriolic and well referenced and documented indignation.

Like the resilient and resourceful rural GPs, I am regularly forced to apply my clinical skills without recourse to other consultant opinions and investigations that are routine in the metropolitan area. Patients and families need answers and decisions on the day, not on the next visit, or after three or four visits when all investigations, consultations, and case conferences have been completed. We are so used to having investigational resources at our finger tips that we have long forgotten that a diagnosis is always clinical in essence.

When I returned to South Australia after gaining a membership of the Royal Colleges of Physicians, MRCP (UK), in the early 1970s, I was the first officially trained Geriatrician in the State. In common with my peers around Australia, I brought with me a keen missionary zeal to introduce Geriatric Medicine into an unwelcoming medico-political environment. I confirmed what I already suspected, that it was extremely difficult to introduce a new specialty into an entrenched system that considered itself state of the art, and was set in concrete.

When healthcare reform is discussed, and this happens around the time of any Commonwealth or State election, the overall shape of the 'system' is taken as a given. It is assumed and accepted that all that is needed to reform 'the best healthcare system in the world' is some minor tinkering with the most visible entities – the hospitals.

To this day, I have very strong feelings about what the shape of the healthcare system should be, and how Geriatric Medicine should be practised. Working in almost complete isolation from the system in the rural and remote regions I have been able, or more precisely had to, implement many of my beliefs and methods.

In summary, I will address the following issues:

- The conventional perception of what Medicine is, the way we perceive illness, and the way we practice does not equip us with a holistic approach. I will argue that there is a schism between the Art and Science of Medicine that must be healed if we are to remain relevant as a profession.

- I contend that this is the era of chronic illness and I will use dementia as the epitome of chronic illness and discuss my beliefs and methods regarding how it, and chronic illness in general, should be addressed.

- I will argue that in the era of super-specialisation Geriatric Medicine is losing its way and raison d'être.

- I will examine how the system and the way that we organise ourselves restricts our approach to clinical care; that the system impedes rather than facilitates the delivery of effective and efficient health care, and that real reform is almost impossible in the current political climate.

- Aged Care is now an oxymoron. It has been labelled as an industry and this is a more honest description of the current reality.

- I will argue that the way we organize ourselves to deliver clinical services increasingly fails to meet the needs of our patient populations.

- There is an urgent need to re-examine our obligations arising from medical and professional ethics. Among other things, we must challenge, not condone the harm that is being done to our patients and their partners and relatives in the name of respect for the 'right' to autonomy.

- I will present a conceptualisation of what dementia is that challenges current orthodoxy.

- I will urge the abandonment and replacement of the term 'dementia'.

- I will argue that the concept of 'patient' must be re-defined in the context of dementia, if not in all chronic illness, and I will prove that it is easier to diagnose dementia accurately without the patient than without the life partner. *This concept is of critical importance in manage-ment and the provision of care.*

- I will outline how assessment, particularly the critical initial assessment of a suspected sufferer from dementia, should be performed.

- I will describe how the patient with a cognitive impairment should be managed in general, and in particular situations, including palliative care.

- Dementia manifests as cognitive impairment. In managing dementia, we give this only minimal and unfocused attention. *Living is learning and every opportunity must be taken to ensure that all activities are designed to train and rehabilitate.*

The Art and Science of Medicine

Art versus Science, or two sides of the same coin?

From inability to let well alone
From too much zeal for the new and contempt for what is old
From putting knowledge before wisdom, science before art, and
Cleverness before common sense;
From treating patients as cases;
And from making the cure of the disease more grievous than
the Endurance of the same,
Good Lord, deliver us.

Sir Robert Hutchison

When I came across this quotation I got very excited because I have always wanted to start a chapter with a quotation.

I dashed off and found my dog-eared copy of *Hutchison's Clinical Methods* by Donald Hunter, R.R. Bomford, 13th edition (1956). The first edition had been dated 1897. In the preface, the authors explained that with the 1956 edition Sir Robert Hutchison retired from active participation in the book.

The purchase of the book was a historic moment in my education as it signalled the beginning of the clinical part of the medical course. No more boring lectures from eminent scientists who had not seemed to have the slightest inkling of the relevance or otherwise of what they taught us to the practice of medicine. This was the real thing, we were going to learn how to become doctors.

It is interesting to note that the debate about the relative merits of the art versus the science is very longstanding. I argue that we have been seduced by what we have chosen to represent as the totality of the Science of Medicine and forsaken the Art. In this critique, I am focusing on what clinicians conventionally accept as the science that underlies the practice of modern medicine.

When I sat for my final MBBS examination in the mid-1960s, one of the examination papers was headed 'The Art and Science of Medicine'. Since then, the Science of Medicine has certainly progressed and is in the ascendant. But what has happened to the Art of Medicine? It seems to have become lost and forgotten. I suspect that many believe that we only needed the Art before we had CTs, MRIs, endoscopies, and easy access to all forms of investigation. Was the Art simply the ability to reach diagnoses equipped only with a stethoscope and percussion hammer because there was nothing better? I think not.

Without wishing to enter into a deep philosophical debate, I think of intelligence as cognitive athleticism. With or without an education, we need it to succeed in life. We also need it to succeed in education as it is currently practised. Those who succeed in education can be construed as cognitive acrobats. They are highly tuned athletes who can succeed in that athletic event known as an examination. I construe intellect as going beyond simple intelligence. I believe that the intellectual individual must have a wide range of interests, imagination, insight, and the capacity to be creative, *in addition* to being able to pass exams.

Doctors believe that they are, de facto, very intelligent, because it is extremely difficult to be accepted into a medical course. This can lead to an assumption that it automatically gives them intellectual superiority over other people. This arrogant assumption gives our profession some of its least endearing characteristics. While giving lip-service to inter-disciplinary cooperation, we nevertheless presume that leadership is our prerogative, and that while we are professionals, the others working alongside us are mere tradesmen or artisans. If the truth be known, in many situations the doctor is the tradesman, and people from other disciplines are the true intellectuals. It is of course possible for doctors to be both intelligent and intellectual. Many are, and history abounds with great examples. Many of these people had been outcasts in their day, and their contribution to the development of Medicine has often been recognised and acknowledged posthumously.

A significant part of the criticism of our profession is the probably, at least historically, correct perception that we have used our privileged position in society to monopolise the provision of valuable services by circumscribing and delegitimising the works of rival practitioners and the knowledge of laypersons, and have restricted the entry of others into our ranks.

In the early debates between the art and science factions within the profession these factions were portrayed as extreme opposites. The art was devalued by being seen as something implicit to the experienced practitioner, and not something that could be codified into rules or learnt by anything other than apprenticeship.

The Science of Medicine – The Medical Model

The 'Medical Model' is at the core of what many clinicians believe constitutes the scientific practice of medicine.

It can be simply summarised as: Symptoms and signs are indicative of an underlying somatic cause that can be identified and then specifically treated, usually with an appropriate medication, or surgically removed.

Implicit in this conceptualisation is that the patient is the person with the pathology. This is *ipso facto* the person that must be diagnosed and treated in order to deal with the presenting manifestations. This is a perception that I will repeatedly challenge in later chapters.

In the 1970s and 1980s the medical model took a battering from its critics. Those on the receiving end were predominantly psychiatrists. They were accused of 'medicalisation'. The main criticism was that normal variations in behaviour, normal physiological, developmental and degenerative processes were too often labelled as diseases in the process of *iatrogenesis* (i.e. any injury or illness that occurs *because of* medical care), for self-serving reasons such as the professional dominance and the exercise of power and control over patients and society in general.

A study of the history of psychiatric nomenclature gives plenty of credence to the idea that psychiatric diagnoses are not nearly as firmly grounded in terms of verifiable science as are somatic diagnoses as we may propose, particularly when we compare them with simple entities such as infectious diseases. We now have DSM-5. It presumably has at least four predecessors, and will continue to have successors, because even with the significant developments in neuroscience, neuropsychology, and functional imaging, the structural changes that underlie psychiatric illnesses do not fully explain the phenomena observed. The release of DSM-5 has been followed by a virtual explosion of critiques as well as publications explaining it and instructing practitioners in its use. I have studied several of each.

Like all polarised debate, those engaged in it hold extreme views. What is 'normal' is in itself a contentious topic. In Medicine, whatever attribute or behaviour we examine, the edges are blurry. We are faced with the bell-shaped curve. A few people are found at either end, and the majority are in the middle. What is a normal blood pressure? In reality there is no clear-cut dividing line between the normal and the abnormal. When does menstruation become a clinical problem? Must every departure from the average norm be stoically accepted as inevitable?

Many disorders are like hypertension, points on a continuum selected for statistical reasons.

Geriatric Medicine has got caught in the crossfire. Ageing and even dementia were included in arguments about medicalisation and iatrogenesis. This has had practical consequences for aged care and has given the opposition an advantage over us in dealings with politicians and the health and welfare bureaucracies.

I can cite numerous examples based on my own experience where attempts at introducing better or even rudimentary medical care and rehabilitation into aged care facilities were resisted as being manifestations of the reprehensible medical model, and its underlying ulterior motivation.

I personally dismiss the perspective that everything that happens in old age is simply a variant of the norm. With dementia, we are talking about a dramatic change that is not an inevitable result of ageing alone and must be due to some form of underlying pathology. There is plenty of pathology to be found that cannot be conveniently classed as 'normal ageing'. However, Dementia sits uncomfortably on the fence between the psychological and the somatic (the psyche and the soma). Despite attempts to define it tightly, as an entity it remains elusive.

The explanation is simple. It is a syndrome. It does not fit comfortably into the medical model conceptualisation in the model's most simplistic form. Once, when frustrated by the beliefs and actions of some of my colleagues I described the medical model as an impenetrable cage built from impervious material. I believe that when adhered to uncritically, it has indeed become a cage, a barrier that limits our thinking and our imagination.

The clinician's concept of what constitutes science has become very concrete. In those distant days when I emerged from medical school, half a century ago, I too was convinced that the science of medicine was indeed based on unquestionable certainty. It is after all made up of concepts, entities, and manifestations that can be seen, measured, and 'proved' to exist. It did not allow for intangibles.

Despite this early faith, as the years have gone by I have found it very difficult to accept the validity of much clinical research and importantly the guidelines based upon it. In reading the history of science, I was somewhat reassured to find that most of the foundations of science have been criticised and questioned for centuries, and while I believe that what we now see is largely valid, there is still room for error and room for doubt. Reading so much philosophical literature has been quite daunting, and I was lucky to find a book by A.F. Chalmers called, *What is this thing called Science?*[*], which made the whole process digestible.

Rather than indulging in displays of righteous indignation, we need to learn from our critics. This does not mean the abandonment of the medical model, but rather accepting and addressing those aspects of the criticism that are valid and re-building a model that is not a cage made from impervious material.

This centres on how we construe the origins of the manifestations (the symptoms and signs) of chronic diseases, and specifically dementia. They cannot be adequately explained with the reductionist view of the

---

* University of Queensland Press, 3rd edn., 1999.

aetiology that was inculcated into us from very early in our medical course.

The categorisation of dementia as a psychiatric illness is also counter-productive. Patients with dementia can suffer from various of the mental illnesses categorised in DSM-5. I also believe that they can suffer significantly from psychological distress that fails to meet the current diagnostic criteria, but nevertheless has to be addressed.

I first met Occam's Razor in the first year of the Medical Course in Biology 1. The Basic Science subjects that we had to accumulate in the preclinical years of the course were taught by scientists who had little understanding of the relevance of science for medical practice. In this instance, the lecturer was a nice man who, unlike some others, took the trouble to make his lectures interesting and entertaining.

It was he who introduced us to Occam's Razor. He worded it as, 'Thou shalt not suppose more causes than are necessary to explain the phenomena observed'. I know that this is what he said because, I like all my contemporaries, took down every word that anybody said, so that we could memorise it, regurgitate it at the next exam, and then try to unclutter our brain with what was mostly irrelevant information. Occam's Razor, however, stayed with me. I subsequently learned that the words above were not those that were uttered by Occam. For a start, the language of science was Latin, and what he is alleged to have said was

Numquam ponenda est pluralitas sine necessitate, which seemed to mean the same thing, although my Latin had become seriously impaired by the time that I found this piece of information.

On arrival in the wards, I discovered that Occam's Razor was alive and well, and living at the Royal Adelaide Hospital. Our clinical teachers believed and taught that Occam's razor, the Law of Parsimony, applied not only in science, but also in clinical practice with regard to diagnosis. You were a bit of a dill if you could not explain all of the manifestations with a single diagnosis. Now, I strongly believe that when confronted by a complex chronic illness, if you think that you can explain all of the manifestations with a simple unitary diagnosis you are worse than a dill, you are dangerously insightless and deluded.

We were also taught the Scientific Method. In a nutshell, it followed a series of steps:

1. Define a question about an issue, a course of action

2. Gather information based on observation

3. Form a hypothesis

4. Test the hypothesis by performing an experiment and gathering the data that arises from it in a manner that could be reproduced by others

5. Analyse that data to determine to what degree it explains the hypothesis and its usefulness and effectiveness in dealing with the issue being addressed, in comparison with doing nothing or undertaking a different course of action.

What results are degrees of probability, and not absolute certainty. Of course, the true scientist recognises that we must have a critical attitude not only towards the theories of others but our own theories as well. Clinical science does not progress to immutable truth. Alas, there are some among us practising medicine who cannot be described as true scientists.

I hasten yet again to assert that I am not a Luddite. I am, however, a sceptic. I believe that we should all be sceptics. For me, the most significant thing about the scientific method is the preparedness to be proved wrong. Ultimately, what differentiates us from the quacks, the charlatans, and even the societally-condoned alternative therapists, is this lack of complete certainty. In an earlier phase of my career, I had a keen interest in peptic ulcers. We were sure that we knew what caused them. That they could be caused by an organism never entered our thinking and would have been considered a crackpot suggestion, if it had been raised at that time. Now thanks to two great Nobel

Prize winning Australian researchers, Barry Marshall and Robin Warren, we know better.

The Science of Medicine – Evidence-based medicine and the Randomised Controlled Trial

The foundation, the gold standard, of the modern clinical scientific method is the Randomised Controlled Trial. I am concerned about the degree with which scientific knowledge acquired by this method is uncritically accepted as infallible and, conversely, anything that falls outside of these parameters is inevitably presumed to be wrong. We are too often left with the conclusion that nothing for which there is no RCT-derived supporting evidence should be done, used or prescribed. Again, one wonders where new ideas will come from.

For the uninitiated, in the conduct of a typical clinical drug trial in the management of a particular condition the objectives and end-points must be clearly defined. The participants who meet the entry criteria are randomly assigned into one of two groups: The Treatment Group or The Placebo Group. This is 'blinded' in that neither the researcher nor the participant knows which group they are in until the end of the trial. All interventions and monitoring are identical in both groups and all the effects and side-effects are recorded identically. The results are subject to sophisticated statistical analysis.

A true sceptic questions everything, not just the assertions of quacks and charlatans, but also the assertions made by our own profession. The unconditional faith in the RCT is the prime example. Over the years, it was painfully clear that old people with comorbidities and cognitive deficits did not meet the entry criteria into drug trials being conducted on agents where they were unquestionably the main target group. This has improved marginally.

The credibility of an RCT depends on very tight definitions of the target problem/issue/manifestation of the intervention, and the outcome. These are only (relatively) easy to define when we are talking about a single clear target indication, e.g. hypertension (however we define it), and we can find people who have it in pure culture. The outcome is very measurable, although the way that we measure it is subject to fluctuations determined by outside factors. For purposes of discussion, let us assume that it is a clear-cut as it appears to be to a non-sceptic.

When the subject is something that is extremely complicated, where many factors impact on the manifestation that is the target for the intervention, let us say dementia, both the manifestation and the outcome are influenced by multiple factors other than the aetiological and pathophysiological assumptions that define the target manifestation.

The outcome is similarly complex, and the actual outcome may be impossible to identify using the blunt instruments available to us. Despite this, what we prescribe and how we intervene is governed by these simplistic, and I contend often meaningless evaluations.

The only instrument that can accurately define the problem in these complex situations and convincingly measure the outcome is the thinking clinician, practising the Art, and not only what we have called the Science of Medicine. This is a particular problem when we subject behavioural and psychological interventions to the structure and assumptions of an RCT.

Our belief in the RCT reaches religious proportions. It is therefore very sobering to look at drugs that have been withdrawn by the FDA, the ultimate arbiter of the efficacy and safety of medication. These are numerous and include many such drugs that were heavily promoted before being withdrawn.

I do not wish to sound dismissive of the contribution that science makes to the way that we practice. Not only has it given us a deep understanding of what we are dealing with, it has also given us structures and methods that enable us to put theory into practice and to monitor and evaluate outcomes. I am arguing against over-certainty and the dismissal of other branches of science outside the biological parameters.

I contend that there is a risk of being too scientific. We are focused on detecting and treating the underlying pathology and pathophysiology (the tangible causes), and we form expectations of what the manifestations can legitimately be. I posit that a specific causal diagnosis is of little value in the clinical situation, especially when there is more than one candidate capable of the pathological damage. We make the symptoms and manifestations reflect the presumed pathology, and do not accept that the manifestations are clinically our prime concern and that our understanding of the pathophysiology may be seriously incomplete.

We close our minds to other possibilities. For example, it is accepted that insight is lost in frontotemporal dementia, and we think that this is in some way linked to the diagnosis. The loss of insight in Alzheimer's disease is seriously under-recognised, and so it may be overlooked as a significant issue, even though it is one of the commonest and most troublesome manifestations that we face.

Not very long ago, many of my colleagues were making confident definitive diagnoses of vascular dementia and concluding that a trial prescription of cholinesterase inhibitor therapy was never indicated. There has now been a complete turnaround in these assumptions.

Transplanting or transferring the way we operate in the research setting into the clinical setting is common, but it is fraught with difficulty. The reasons that subjects enter into a trial are different from the reasons that patients present to their clinician. The relationship that they enter into is not the classical clinical doctor–patient relationship. The assessment that they undergo is highly focused and not generalised into other aspects of the patient's life and functioning.

I have participated in drug trials and this has been a valuable experience for me. Not the least of which was gaining familiarity with numerous assessment instruments. Unlike some others, I have not patterned my clinical practice on the way that I contributed to the trial. One of the most lasting lessons, however, was learning how difficult it was to find people who met the inclusion criteria, and how little resemblance there ultimately was between the trial participants and the people that I see in everyday practice.

I have regularly had to defend colleagues, when patients and relatives have complained that they were very dissatisfied with the way that they were treated in the course of a drug trial. I pointed out that the colleagues concerned had private practices and were highly respected in the profession and by their patients, and that their behaviour and relationship with the patient was very different between settings. I too have been the provider of the physician's input in trials, while other people dealt with other issues, and were like me, bit players and not soloists as any of us would have been in the ordinary clinical setting.

I am frequently asked to resolve behavioural issues in residential care facilities. I always interview as many care staff as are available on the occasion. Within a few minutes, I can predict, almost infallibly, which carers are likely to have had difficulty dealing with the subject behaviour, and those who have not, based on my impression of their personalities and attitudes, irrespective of their level of training. How do you design a trial that can randomly allocate residents into groups that have similar characteristics, and then study the intervention and define and measure a meaningful outcome in a totally uncontrollable setting?

The Science without the Art can be robotic. Alas, I can think of colleagues to whom that description could be aptly applied. Computers could be programmed to diagnose and prescribe for conditions which best fit the definitions fed into them. However, most if not all of these definitions are subject to debate and must be interpreted by a capable practitioner to determine if they apply. I will deal with psychiatric diagnosis in a later chapter.

A lot of research is based on the use of screening instruments. These are also used to save time and effort in trials. I have been able to compare well-validated instruments screening for dementia, depression, anxiety and carer stress with my own face-to-face interviews. Most of the time these tests indicate that there is an issue but cannot stand alone as being diagnostic. At times, they are completely misleading, and if one relied on their validity very important issues would be missed.

I know many intelligent, well-informed people as friends, patients, carers and relatives, who prefer the assistance of alternative practitioners. When questioned, they express dissatisfaction with the way that they have been treated by conventional medical practitioners. They were not given time and were subjected to tests that they did not understand to be relevant to their predicament: 'The doctor took away dad's licence because he couldn't spell the word "world" backwards.'

They did not receive explanations that were comprehensible (the amyloid cascade is of limited interest to the average person) and did not sound as plausible as the pseudoscience of the alternative practitioner. Treatment was offered in ways that failed to instil confidence and raised the fear of adverse effects: 'These drugs may help a bit in a small percentage of patients. Oh, and I need to tell you that there is a very remote risk of stroke.'

Elements of the Art of Medicine

The Art of Medicine comprises the intellectual, cognitive and emotional qualities that the clinician can bring to bear. This sounds awfully like interpersonal skills. The Art enables the clinician to see the Science in a broad perspective and to apply it with the recognition of its strengths and weaknesses.

Ultimately, irrespective of the guidelines, algorithms, instruments and gimmicks at our disposal, our decisions and interventions must be essentially clinical. It is our clinical acumen and judgement that will be questioned and challenged if there are adverse outcomes for our patients, and not our ability to debate the statistical significance of the findings in an RCT.

If our clinical behaviour or judgement is questioned, the best defence is a clinical record that accurately describes the proceedings and offers clear evidence of the reasoning that led to our conclusions and subsequent actions.

As I have argued above, scepticism is, almost by definition, an essential requirement in the make-up of the true scientist. That is why medicine needs its iconoclasts. Without scepticism, we can be accused of being as guilty of pseudoscience as the alternative practitioners we disregard.

I set out with a fairly simple understanding (belief?) of what constitutes the Art of Medicine. I began with a few key words, describing attributes, qualities, abilities etc. As I examined each of them, additional words and concepts came to light. To a degree, many are self-evident and I will therefore list the words and concepts and only expand on some of them.

Personal attributes

Qualities and Capacities

Humanity

Open-mindedness

Trustfulness

Tolerance

Objectivity

Impartiality and Fairness

Sympathy

Empathy

Intuition

Reasoning

Judgement

Abilities

Establishing rapport, trust

Communication

Observation

Defusing hostility and aggression

Reducing anxiety

Education

Counselling

I believe that the Art of Medicine can and should be taught just like the Science. It is the intellectual part of medicine. While the way we acquire these characteristics is strongly based on personal experience, it is important to realise that they are highly definable and highly studied topics. We should realise that there are many branches of psychology, sociology, education, and other humanistic and behavioural sciences that have long been scientific in their methods. In other words, the Art of Medicine is science-based.

Observation is something that we are all capable of, but not everyone uses. A biblical quote (paraphrased no doubt, but it gained something in the translation) comes to mind: 'See and you see, but you do not perceive; hear and you hear, but you do not understand.'

Observation is simple to teach. In a medical course we learn palpation and auscultation, among many skills that call for the use of our senses and accept that this yields information that will aid us in arriving at a diagnosis. There are many other ways in which we can use our senses.

When I undertake a home visit with a student, as we get out of the car I say, 'Turn on your brain. The consultation has started. Everything that you see, hear, smell or feel from now on is important information.' We note that our patient lives in a good neighbourhood, but that her house is badly in need of maintenance. Her front garden is a jumble of weeds. Her gate does not close properly. The gravel path to her front door is loose and uneven. There are two steps up to the veranda where her front door is. There is a bad smell even before we enter the house. The door is securely locked with a dead lock. The doorbell does not work and we have to knock loudly to attract attention.

We have acquired all this valuable and very relevant information even before we set eyes on the patient. I have been doing home visits since time immemorial, but it was working with Occupational Therapists that taught me how a home visit should really be conducted in a systematic manner.

When the Problem Oriented Medical Record was introduced into a hospital where I was then a medical registrar, several respected senior clinicians protested, as they were unable to explain and document how they reached their conclusions, the process being so intuitive.

Intuition may be construed in many different ways. I think of it as dredging the morass of unrelated data that is my memory, and then making a connection with the situation at hand.

I have always been curious and an avid and voracious reader. I cannot have breakfast without reading the cereal packet, the label on the jam jar, or anything else that is printed. When I eat in hotels by myself I bring a book. My mind is full of seemingly useless facts, although I am a useful team member at Quiz nights.

Often when I look at a situation, everything suddenly falls into place. I think that what happens is analogous to using an internet search engine. Seemingly unrelated facts turn out to be not only related but relevant. I too would have difficulty explaining how I arrived at my conclusion. An interesting observation is how often something that has been eluding me seems very clear in the morning. Writing this book has seriously impinged on my life. I get unexpected inspirations in the shower, doing my exercise, on the plane, waiting for the dentist et cetera that are so clear that they must be immediately jotted down. The process is akin to retrieving procedural memory in its subconscious way.

If I had to find somewhere to put intuition into a box, I would include it as an example of executive function.

I am sure that all advanced trainees, and probably many senior students, have more factual knowledge and scientific understanding than I do. Despite this, I feel that I am a much more effective clinician than I was when I was the advanced trainee who knew so much more factual information than my clinical mentors and teachers.

What I have is vast experience and insights that are not found in textbooks. I have the confidence to make decisions and diagnoses that seem at odds with the conventional wisdom. In my final year in medical school I attended no formal lectures because I felt that I could read as well as the clinical teachers who simply regurgitated what was in the set texts. What they did not do in that context was teach me the tricks of the trade, which they knew and that I did not.

Therefore, instead of attending lectures I read voraciously and haunted the casualty departments and wards of our teaching hospitals. I gained my best academic results in the final year exams. That is a lesson I have never forgotten.

As an aside, while the 'tricks of the trade' may not be found in text books, they can be taught by apprenticeship. I am opposed to the Ward Round as a teaching venue and method. It can be demeaning and does not do justice to patients. Clinicians can only demonstrate their mechanical and intellectual, rather than truly clinical, skills. For some, it is simply a theatrical ego trip.

I prefer to be accompanied by a single student or trainee while I do a case-taking. I try not to see people at the bedside in a multi-bed ward but sit, face-to-face with the patient in a quiet, private setting. Most will accept a single observer but are intimidated by a crowd. I always ask permission for the student to attend. If the permission is refused for any reason the patient's wishes are honoured. Most patients agree and are indeed eager to help the student to learn.

Like no doubt most of my colleagues, I see myself as a perpetual student. I try to keep up to date on all of the areas within which I practise, and my reports to general practitioners are researched to ensure that my advice and recommendations are in keeping with current best practice. My reports are also structured so that it is clear on what evidence and by what reasoning I reached my conclusions and recommendations.

Long ago, one of my clinical mentors taught me to consider whether I could defend what I had written in a court of law, should that need arise. I always offer evidence for what I say, conclude and recommend. That is not to say that I am always right, and that I cannot be proved wrong. It simply means that the recipient of my report can follow the reasoning that went into it and judge the quality of the evidence that I offer for himself. As a Geriatrician, I make numerous decisions that can be classed 'medico-legal' and they are regularly put to the legal test. I never label my reports 'Not to be used for medico-legal purposes' as most of my psychiatric colleagues seem to do, because I have no fear that anything I say can be successfully used against me.

When I teach at any level, I point out that I will focus on clinical skills and reasoning, rather than providing factual information. I relent somewhat with more junior students by giving them prepared handouts on the topic that they thought was going to be addressed in my teaching session. With more senior students, I tell them how to find the information and encourage them to do their own research and then share their findings with me and their fellow students. Over the years I've learnt a great deal by this method. Increasingly, today's students are better able to tell me how to find the relevant information.

We have paid a price for this explosive burgeoning of new information. In self-defence, we have organised ourselves into specialties, subspecialties, sub- sub-specialties, ad infinitum. An aphorism attributed to Mahatma Ghandi summarises this point: 'The expert knows more and more about less and less until he knows everything about nothing.'

We have almost lost the generalists. I vividly remember when the teaching hospital I was working in at the time dismissed the General Physicians and made the Specialist Units responsible for the take-in system. Several of these general physicians offered themselves to the Geriatric Unit, the last post for generalists. I did not have the funding to accommodate them, and they drifted into the private hospital system, where some continue to this day providing an excellent essential clinical service. Even general practitioners have to sub-specialise.

This super-specialisation enables us to deal very effectively with clear-cut diseases and disorders. I would not be alive today to write these words were it not for super-specialists to whom I am eternally grateful. The weakness is in the inability to effectively manage syndromes. In hospitals, the risk is that without the effective triage that a skilled generalist can provide, a patient can be streamed into the wrong specialty sometimes with disastrous consequences.

I have been bewailing the passing of the Art of Medicine. A more worrying reality is that it is assumed that those among us who obviously excel in the Science, must also excel in the Art. Thus, it follows that an outstanding researcher is also an outstanding clinician, teacher and health administrator. Ask yourself the question: How many people have you met who meet all these specifications?

Summation

Our belief in what we conventionally construe as science has become dogma. I remind the reader that dogma is a set of principles laid down by an authority and is deemed by the adherents of that authority as incontrovertibly true. We perceive our version of science as dogma. This orthodoxy closes our minds.

In the context of dementia, we think that we now know what cognitive function is and what the diagnostic features of dysfunction are. We certainly know a vast amount more about cognitive function than we knew in the 1970s, when the Mini Mental State Examination was introduced by Folstein. How scientific is it to accept that an MMSE score is absolute evidence of the presence or absence of dementia, and furthermore that it is a meaningful measure of severity? I regularly see examples of respected neurologists, psychiatrists and geriatricians afflicted with this delusional belief.

When I have questioned this, it has been pointed out to me that it is a well validated test and has been the chosen test in numerous scientific tests and trials right up to the present day. I ask the question, 'Validated against what?' Whatever they choose to say, the reality is that it is based on a conceptualisation of dementia that has not progressed for fifty years. It goes with the tacit acceptance that the onset dates from the time of diagnosis, and we must invent entities like Mild Cognitive Impairment to kill time before making a confident diagnosis that meets current diagnostic criteria, often in the context of a crisis in the patient's life. Again, this is also something that I see regularly, and could produce many examples from my records if pressed.

Similarly, the Frontal Assessment Battery is often deemed to tell us all we need to know about executive function.

Neuropsychology has made dramatic advances, but there is a great deal that we still do not know with certainty. The findings from even the most sophisticated tests currently available must be interpreted. Most definitions of dementia focus on memory as the critical functional entity, without changes in which the diagnosis of dementia is not tenable.

I remind the reader that clinically-related science is applied science. Scientific findings, however abstruse, must always be interpreted in the current context, which is always by its very nature unique. The finding must be translated, transferred into everyday reality and relevance for the people at the centre of the clinical situation, which I posit is the patient and the life-partner/relative/key carer. This cannot be done without the application of what I have described as the art.

M.D. Lezak,[*] whose scientific credentials are beyond reproach, writing on volition as a component of executive function, makes the following observation: '… there are no formal tests for examining volitional capacity. The examiner must rely instead on observations of these patients in the normal course of day-to-day living and reports by caregivers, family, and others who see them regularly.'

There are a number of critically important manifestations of dementia that can only be elicited by skilled interview of the patient and the life-partner/relative.

The assessor must not only interpret the simple test result but extrapolate beyond, into its meaning in the present predicament and in the future.

Amongst the clinical sciences, my favourite is Occupational Therapy. It is the prime example of applying science to every aspect of everyday life.[†]

[*]   Lezak M.D., Howieson D.B. & Loring D.W., *Neuropsychological Assessment,* Oxford University Press, 4th edn., 2004, p. 612.

[†]   Gillen G., *Cognitive and Perceptual Rehabilitation*, Mosby Inc, 2009.

Research, as epitomised by the RCT drug trial, has come to dominate the practice of Medicine. The goals, methods and reasoning of research and one-on-one clinical care are related, but far from identical.

The group of experts gathered together for a multinational drug trial is not a clinical team. The relationship between the participating physician and the subject is not a true clinical relationship. The clinician's goals are to fulfil his obligations to the patient in this clinical predicament, in the here and now.

Thus, the Art and Science of Medicine are like two sides of a coin, one is incomplete without the other. It is like going through life deprived of half of our senses. If we lack the insight and do not know any better, we assume that we are whole. Simply put, the science without the art is like a body without a soul.

In every clinical situation, all information must be critically analysed and interpreted in the context before it is applied.

The Art fleshes out the science and takes it from the laboratory to the outside world. It enables us to find the relevance of the findings highly of focused neuropsychological research and extrapolate how they explains some clinical phenomenon in ways that we have not previously considered.

It allows us to take a wide (versus microscopic) view and recognise the significance of findings and interventions in other related fields and apply them to the issues that confront us.

It takes management beyond pharmacotherapy and enables us to find alternative ways of managing our patients and those who share their predicament.

Words with power

Evidence-based. The ascendancy of the conventional view of the Science of Medicine dominates how we teach, organise, practise medicine and measure and judge the quality of what we do. By adhering to guidelines, the dogma based on what we construe is the appropriate evidence, we can satisfy ourselves that we do well.

When reading about theories and models of cognitive disorders in the psychological literature, the following statement is not uncommon: 'None of these hypotheses can explain the experimental data entirely' – but they can explain issues encountered in a clinical situation.

In clinical medicine, the ultimate measure of quality is the outcome of the one-on-one clinical consultation, remembering that we are dealing with people who are affected by the manifestations of a disorder and are suffering.

From the patient's and partner's perspective, quality means that the presenting concerns, complaints and distress have been addressed, explained and resolved.

In the diagnosis/assessment of a suspected sufferer of dementia in accordance with current best-practice criteria it is not just possible, but highly probable, that the presenting concerns will not even have been detected, and certainly not have been resolved, in any way.

2

Conceptualising Dementia

Dementia epitomises *chronic* illness. It has many dimensions and no special field of knowledge, including Psychiatry, owns it, though many specialties have contributed to our understanding of it and continue to play a very important role in its management. Psychiatry and Neurology have led in the acquisition of knowledge. Pathology, Radiology, Genomics and others have also made dramatic contributions to what we know and do. However, questions remain as to who should perform the initial clinical assessment and manage the patient with dementia from day-to-day.

These questions become ever more pertinent when we look at how most of the conventional specialties have splintered in many directions, becoming more and more focused on detail, and further and further away from a generalist perspective and capability.

The fact that several quite diverse specialties may claim dementia as their natural preserve should alert us to the probability of doubts about the degree to which there is consensual agreement as to the fundamental nature of the process of dementia and how it should be treated.

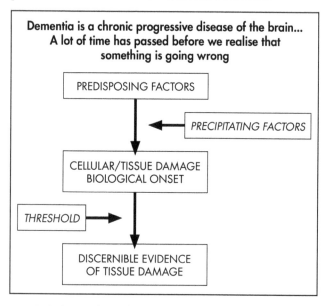

**Dementia is a chronic progressive disease of the brain...
A lot of time has passed before we realise that
something is going wrong**

PREDISPOSING FACTORS

PRECIPITATING FACTORS

CELLULAR/TISSUE DAMAGE
BIOLOGICAL ONSET

THRESHOLD

DISCERNIBLE EVIDENCE
OF TISSUE DAMAGE

I believe that dementia is a chronic progressive neurodegenerative disease of the brain that is severely disabling and ultimately fatal. It can also result from any illness or injury that damages the brain extensively. In common with all diseases, there are predisposing and precipitating factors that lead to the pathological damage that will eventually result in a syndrome, a complex combination of signs, symptoms and dysfunction that goes beyond the cognitive damage alone. As in most chronic diseases, both the predisposing and precipitating causes are multifactorial. In dementia, it is highly probable that quite some time has passed before the interaction of those predisposing and precipitating factors results in manifestations that can be identified and hence diagnosed.

To date, we have tended to equate the onset of dementia with the first appearance of cognitive change. This is rather like assuming that coronary artery disease begins with the onset of angina or a myocardial infarction.

In the pathological development of the disease, and thereafter, there is a series of thresholds when the damage, first at a sub-cellular level, then a cellular level, then at tissue level, gives opportunities to discern and measure *change from the pre-existing state* or from what is normal in the individual. This is followed by other thresholds that can be identified with increasing ease.

In the development of diagnostic criteria, we have chosen one of the late thresholds as signalling the time of onset of the disease. This is in keeping with our conventional way of practising medicine. We recognise the illness by its symptoms and signs and we deal with episodes at an instant in time, not an entire disease process, in a continuum.

Later in the book I seriously question the validity of current methods and assumptions in the diagnostic assessment process. Any thought of early diagnosis based on more sophisticated cognitive testing is, however, a pipedream: diagnosis based on current and similar criteria will always be late. Unfortunately, by then the window of opportunity to intervene effectively in a preventive–or therapeutic manner may long have closed.

Diseases damage tissues...

Damage in tissues leads to...

- Symptoms – what the patient experiences
- Signs – what can be observed or elicited
- Impairment & Loss of that tissue's function that can be demonstrated & measured

---

Diseases damage tissues. The results of that tissue damage enable us to identify and diagnose the underlying condition. The brain is a tissue. It is however the most complex tissue in the body and it has a multiplicity of functions. Nevertheless, dementia can be understood by patients and relatives if explained in this way. It can be likened to something simple, such as arthritis of the knee. The patient experiences pain and presents to a doctor with this problem. The doctor can examine the knee and find deformity, signs of inflammation, and so on. The patient's walking is affected, and limitation of movement can be demonstrated, measured and documented. It interferes with the patient's ability to work and enjoy social participation.

All of this also happens when the tissue that is damaged is the brain. All manifestations can be attributed to damage to the brain, and ultimately, to a large degree but never completely, to specific areas within the brain. The damage that occurs in all forms of dementia is generally patchy and not localised with pinpoint accuracy, because very complex networks and systems of interconnection further complicate localisation. The loss of connections distant from the area of functional localisation can mean the loss of that function without the loss of the specific cells.

Our medical model obsession with precise definition, hence identification of the growing number of 'specific' types of dementia that are emerging, can close our eyes to features that are present in all forms, but may be ignored because they do not fit the expected pattern of a diagnostic entity as currently defined.

Again, many of us, guided by complete faith in the diagnostic criteria that are in vogue, may fail to look beyond the narrow range of manifestations that are included among the diagnostic criteria. Many never ask the question, 'Is that all there is?' Does the condition that we have diagnosed as defined adequately explain the situation that we see before us and equip us to intervene meaningfully?

For me, the 1980 WHO publication *International Classification of Impairments, Disabilities, and Handicaps* was very exciting, as it gave us a language for conceptualising and classifying and even the capability to measure the consequences of illness, within a sequence:

Disease -> Impairment -> Disability -> Handicap

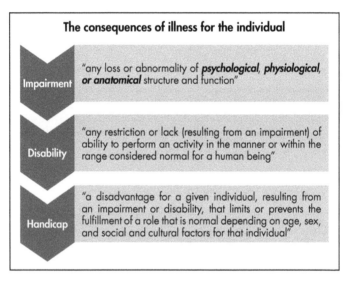

The consequences of illness for the individual

Impairment
"any loss or abnormality of *psychological, physiological, or anatomical* structure and function"

Disability
"any restriction or lack (resulting from an impairment) of ability to perform an activity in the manner or within the range considered normal for a human being"

Handicap
"a disadvantage for a given individual, resulting from an impairment or disability, that limits or prevents the fulfillment of a role that is normal depending on age, sex, and social and cultural factors for that individual"

An *impairment* was defined as 'any loss or abnormality of psychological, physiological, or anatomical structure and function' (i.e. the structural and physiological consequence). In this context, we focus on the pathological causes of dementia. We make distinctions between cortical and sub cortical. Simply put whether the brunt of the damage is with nerve cells or the connections between cell bodies. This is important, but it should not close our eyes to the things that all dementias have in common, with the implication that therapeutic and rehabilitative interventions directed at one sub-type of dementia may be applicable to all.

A *disability* was defined as 'any restriction or lack (resulting from an impairment) of ability to perform an activity in the manner or within the range considered normal for a human being' (i.e. the functional consequence). The function that is unique to the brain is cognitive function. In analysing the functional consequences of cognitive impairment, we must examine each cognitive function in detail in order to understand the extent of the disability in real-life terms. I will deal with this in greater detail in the chapter on the Initial Assessment.

Dementia continues to be thought of as predominantly a memory disorder. Far too many practitioners believe that a simple screening test, such as the MMSE (the Mini Mental State Examination, perhaps the most commonly used screening test to this day) can not only conclusively diagnose or dismiss dementia, but also measure its severity. However, the cardinal feature of dementia is not memory loss: it is the *progressive loss of executive function*.

The loss of executive function has, unfortunately, been presented as the diagnostic feature of frontotemporal and related dementias, with only passing reference to Alzheimer's disease. I believe that this is a failure of diagnostic methodology, and not a true reflection of the actual circumstances.

The disability due to dementia is largely the result of cognitive damage, and in particular the loss of executive function. Our efforts at rehabilitation must be based on this premise. This is not to say that the main causal disease cannot itself cause disability that is not cognitively based; nor that comorbidities almost certainly contribute to the disability that we see. In all cases, the cognitive losses will, however, significantly affect rehabilitative potential.

A *handicap* was defined as 'a disadvantage for a given individual, resulting from an impairment or a disability that limits or prevents the fulfilment of a role that is normal (depending on age, sex, and social and cultural factors) for that individual' (the social consequence). Yes, I am aware of later editions of this publication, but they do not alter the usefulness of the lessons that I learnt from the original.

Again, the handicap has many causes. Some of these require medical intervention. I refer particularly to anxiety, which I contend is an almost universal psychiatric feature of dementia.

Cognitive impairment has an impact on behaviour, emotion, and the capacity of the patient to make and maintain relationships and adapt to social situations.

What the clinician must always keep in mind is that they are dealing with an individual who has undergone deleterious change in their level of functioning. We are not dealing with developmental or intellectual disability. Our patient had considerable life experience and had been functioning generally at a much higher level before the emergence of the neurodegenerative process. That person had beliefs, values, attitudes, strategies and patterns of behaviour in response to many life situations. The essence of diagnosis in dementia is the recognition and demonstration of these changes.

It must also always be kept in mind that the impairment, the disability and the handicap are all present to varying degrees whenever we see the patient and can be clearly identified and even measured. They must then be addressed simultaneously for management to be completely appropriate and effective.

Illness in general, and dementia in particular, is a major threat to the independence and autonomy of elderly people, and in Geriatric Medicine many of our efforts are rightly directed towards the prevention and alleviation of disability and handicap, rather than the causes of the impairment. This is seen as right and proper, indeed so obvious that it does not need saying, when we are dealing with the other great cause of damage to brains – strokes.

There is growing evidence that rehabilitation is feasible in the face of cognitive impairment. I am not referring to the myriad of quaintly named interventions offered by alternative therapists, even though they may be quite effective because of the sincerity and good intent of the practitioners. I commend the book *Cognitive and Perceptual Rehabilitation* by Glenn Gillen, which showed me that this belief in rehabilitation for those with dementia is based on scientific reality.

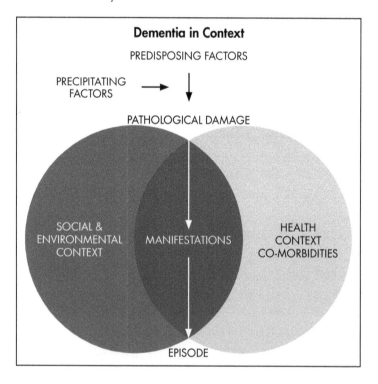

I am regularly asked to explain why assessment of dementia sufferers is not a waste of time and effort when 'we can't treat it'. The answer is simple, there are many things that we can and should do beyond prescribing medication. Indeed, prescribing something is often the worst thing that we can do. There is more to the practice of medicine than applied pharmacology.

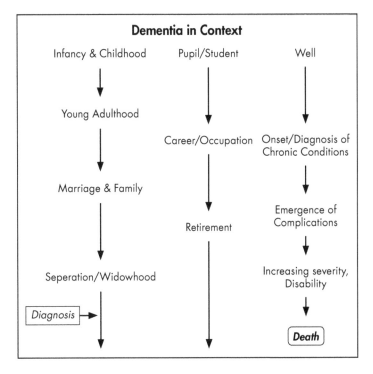

In developed countries we entered the era of *chronic illness* some time ago without giving the phenomenon its due recognition. Chronic illnesses have many significant and important differences from acute illness. All chronic illnesses have many, various attributes. We need to be aware that what we are seeing is a snapshot of an instant in a lifeline, and the disease will progress and will continue to be affected by many more things, some predictable, and some not. There is nothing simple about natural history.

The disease process has its own natural history, but it occurs and develops in the context of comorbidities (also known as multimorbidity, a list that grows with age) that may cause, exacerbate or modify the manifestations that present to us. The treatment of the disease and comorbidities may add to the complexity of the presentation.

When we see a complex presentation, such as delirium, we commonly talk about everyone being different and unique, but we still approach it as an abstract entity, and fail to deal with it as something that is unique to this individual, at this time, in this situation.

To recapitulate, an acute episode of a chronic illness happens in a context. It is a brief event in the course of a very long timeline. Another perspective is however possible, and that is to see the disease in the context of the path of personal development, occupation and health.

Let us look briefly at how we perceive Type II

Diabetes. We have a very serious chronic disease whose origins are much clearer and better understood than those of dementia, but where there is still room for speculation and further research. Its total manifestations are not entirely explicable by the pathology of the pancreas. This becomes increasingly so when complications appear, even though the pathology of each of these complications is also reasonably well understood. The clinician who understands most about the primary pathology, the endocrinologist, can no longer claim to be the ultimate expert on how to manage the complications, and must be prepared to consult with, and ultimately leave the definitive management to those whose area of expertise it is, while still retaining an overview. In a real-life situation, the general practitioner, rather than the endocrinologist or any other specialist, has an overview of the patient in total context. Everyone accepts this. In the case of dementia, however, this logical and automatic recognition that other forms of expertise are required does not necessarily follow, and there is a tendency to perceive it as 'belonging' to a specialty, be it Neurology or Psychiatry, from go to whoa.

Many physicians, excellent in their own fields, have little understanding of what other specialties and disciplines, such as Nursing and the Allied Health Professions, actually do and can achieve. They may not know how to behave in an interdisciplinary mode. 'We have a great team … They do exactly what I tell them.'

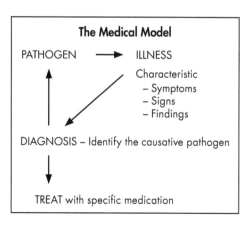

The Medical Model

PATHOGEN ⟶ ILLNESS

Characteristic
– Symptoms
– Signs
– Findings

DIAGNOSIS – Identify the causative pathogen

TREAT with specific medication

Dementia is, though, quite unlike the illnesses we are used to dealing with. Our assumptions, based on the simple medical model, do not adequately explain what is happening to the patient, nor why it is happening.

In dementia, irrespective of which version we try to diagnose, it should become obvious that all of the current manifestations that we see cannot be attributed to a discrete single cause explained from a strict medical model perspective, and this is because we are dealing with a *syndrome* and not a simple illness. Most of the manifestations cannot be defined tightly enough to make them sufficiently strictly measurable to use them as targets for intervention in RCTs. (The Randomised Controlled Trial is the current gold standard in trials of mainly pharmacological interventions where every element can be tightly defined.)

As a syndrome, dementia is a complex condition that extends not only to the disease itself, but also to common presentations of it that impede successful management. Disturbed behaviour, the commonest and most difficult complication to live with and to manage, must also be seen from this perspective, as I will discuss later.

The rigid application of the medical model is not enough. Diagnosing a discrete form of dementia and treating the presumed underlying pathophysiological cause pharmacologically will be of little value to the patient and to the patient's life partner, family and carers. By the time the disease presents our available drugs are of little value in reversing, alleviating or even slowing the progression of the disease. What makes dementia a problem is the disability *and* the behavioural, functional and social consequences of that pathology. This combination of factors is seldom or only partially responsive to therapies designed to alter the course of the pathological damage that causes the disease.

But... Dementia is a Syndrome not a simple disease

All of the manifestations can not be explained by a single pathological process

---

I contend that dementia is the most disabling illness that we are confronted by. The significance of this fact is only vaguely understood because we may be faced by a patient who seems physically intact and capable of normal motor function ('I know she can do it, I've seen her do it if I stand over her …'). Despite this, the patient becomes progressively incapable of living independently. She does poorly on all measures of the basic and instrumental activities of daily living, yet we fail to make the intellectual connection to the cause of that disability and understand that our intervention must focus on it as a problem that must be managed. Looked at in this light, dementia can readily be shown to be more disabling than a severe stroke. The stroke sufferer will adapt to the disability even if actual recovery is limited and will be able to enlist her social and family resources in a useful way. The dementia sufferer will deteriorate inexorably and will resist rather than enlist support.

We should also be aware that the handicap that the dementia sufferer faces. The patient's behaviour leads to the fracturing of key relationships, misunderstanding, discrimination and social stigma. The way that the dementia sufferer is perceived in their capacity to do things and make decisions is seriously affected. As someone who has done many care assessments in hospitals I believe that those that bear that label are treated quite different particularly if delirium is part of their presentation.

Revisiting the second childhood

'Descending into her *second childhood.*' This term has generally been seen as pejorative. Synonyms include such terms as *dotage* and *senility.*

The similarity of what may give parents difficulty with managing the behaviour of their children, and what they may face with their parent reveals striking similarities.

In my readings and observations, and listening to what partners and relatives were saying, I have observed in particular that what was found in ADHD (Attention Deficit Hyperactivity Disorder) and SMD (Sensory Modulation Disorder) was clearly happening at the other end of the age spectrum. Both phenomena form a big part of the behavioural disturbance seen in dementia. The research, the understanding and the management of both by practitioners of many disciplines, including education, occupational therapy and the clinical specialties of paediatrics and psychiatry, is light years ahead of what is happening at the old age end of the spectrum.

There is a lesson here. When we conceptualise, we must take a broad longitudinal perspective. What the paediatrician faces in dealing with problems in the development of cognitive functions and capacities, the Geriatricians face with the decline of the same functions and capacities – the reverse of development, but the manifestations are similar and our attempts at intervention should be informed by the advances made at the other end of the spectrum.

The approach that I have taken throughout this book is a variation on the Bio-Psycho-Social model developed by a psychiatrist, George Engel.*

Approaching any chronic illness any other way is irrational and doomed to fail.

Summation

- Dementia is a chronic, progressive neuro-degenerative disease. It can also be caused by any disease or injury that causes extensive brain damage.

- It begins when a predisposed individual is affected by a triggering cause of pathological damage, a precipitating pathogen.

- The pathology of the disease begins at a cellular level and progresses until there is sufficient damage to be reflected in abnormalities of structure and function of

---

* Engel G, 'The need for a new medical model: a challenge for bio-medicine', *Science,* 1977, 196: 129–36. See also a review by Francesc Borrell-Carrió, Anthony L. Suchman, Ronald M. Epstein clarifies Engels work: *The Biopsychosocial Model 25 Years Later: Principles, Practice, and Scientific Inquiry.*

some part of the tissue of the brain.

- The pathological damage increases progressively and there are a series of thresholds that enable the structural and functional manifestations of this damage to be detected.

- This progression continues after the damage has resulted in a definable clinical illness characterised by what I call the manifestations of the damage: the signs, symptoms, behavioural, personality and emotional changes and the disability.

- The damage that is unique to the brain is cognitive impairment. The crucial cognitive impairment in dementia is not memory loss, but loss of executive function.

- This is happening to an individual who is also progressively ageing, and has comorbidities, several of which may also be progressive.

- The comorbidities strongly affect the disease's presentation, and I believe that any condition that can damage neurones and their connections *can per se* contribute directly to the cognitive impairment.

- *Is mixed dementia the new norm?* At times a clear diagnosis of the type of dementia cannot be made and I believe that mixed dementia is quite common.

- By the time that the diagnosis is made by current methods, the disease has been progressing for a considerable time.

- At presentation for medical attention the disease must be seen in its context from a longitudinal, not just from a cross-sectional, perspective. It is very important that the comorbidities are also considered in the same way.

- The essence of diagnosis in dementia is the recognition and demonstration of changes in cognitive capacity, independent function, behaviour, and the ability to adapt to change.

- This applies not only to the impairment, but also the resulting disability, and the handicap that is faced by the patient. Dementia is a progressively disabling illness.

- Dementia cannot be said to be properly managed unless all of the presenting manifestations have been addressed in some way.

- Dementia is fatal.

A critical part of conceptualisation is understanding that dementia does not just afflict the individual who is affected by the pathology, it afflicts a relationship: the patient and the life-partner, relative, or key carer, who is directly affected by the consequences of the dementia and may be doing more of the 'suffering' and carrying a greater burden than 'the patient'. See also the Initial Assessment section, when cognitive screening and instruments are discussed.

Last lingering thought on early diagnosis

Earlier diagnosis is already possible. I do it all the time. Our obsession with the MMSE score as a valid determining factor of the presence or absence of dementia, and as the way we conventionally conduct initial assessments, closes our minds. I address this in detail in the Initial Assessment section. The key is in understanding that Dementia afflicts a relationship, not just an individual.

The numbers of people with high MMSE scores that I have confidently diagnosed with dementia runs into at least many hundreds. Because I have been visiting some communities for 30–40 years I have a longitudinal perspective on my diagnostic accuracy. I have found many people with high MMSE scores not to have decision-making capacity, and my evidence has been accepted by the former Guardianship Board, and now the Civil and Administrative Tribunal. These are judicial tribunals that base decisions on the quality of the evidence presented to them.

What's in a name?

- We act the way we think
- Our thinking can be guided or constrained by the acceptance of concepts
- Specialisation can be constricting when a degree of generalisation is needed to see the whole picture
- Labels can harm the patient and close our minds

I have also seen many people reluctantly diagnosed with Mild Cognitive Impairment by other consultants present with a crisis just weeks or months later, when dementia is not only diagnosable, but severe. One wonders how many people are never referred by general practitioners because the patient scores well on the MMSE, yet partners and families have serious doubts about that person's capacity, and the reasons that they sought an assessment have not been explained or addressed.

If a marker, most probably genetic, is found, early in the progression of the neuropathology, that predicts a high probability that the person will go on to develop a dementia, shall be faced with a significant ethical dilemma, unless we can offer effective prevention or treatment.

Words with power

Dementia. In this scientific era, this a strange word to describe several diseases that that can be grouped under much more precise and less deprecatory headings. It is from Latin: dementia: 'madness, insanity', literally 'being out of one's mind'. Synonyms for dementia include such words as 'mental decay', 'insanity', 'madness', 'lunacy' and 'derangement'. It is often used in a pejorative sense and is offensive and demeaning.

In my experience patients are terrified of the label, and the term 'Alzheimer's disease' now also evokes very similar responses and carries an identical stigma.

The word has been on the euphemism treadmill (a wonderful term introduced by the cognitive scientist Steven Parker) which describes the progression of a bland euphemism into a slur and an insult.

I suggest we adopt the term *Neuro-Degenerative Disorder* (NDD) or *Neuro-Cognitive Disorder* (NCD, as in DSM-5). What could be less offensive and more difficult to evolve into a form of defamation?

Context. The context within which all medical or behavioural issues present and are addressed is always of critical importance. The context, including not only the degree of dementia but also all comorbidities, the social situation, and the care setting, always determines how management should be approached, and the balance between risks and benefits that must be maintained. It should always be kept in mind. One guideline does not fit all.

3

Ethical Issues

I consider this to be the most important chapter of this book. All else that I say hinges on it.

In the modern era, medical ethics is a wide concept. To be true to our profession we doctors are obliged to act ethically at all times, not only as practitioners but also as members of professional organisations, and members of society and citizens of our country.

Dementia is by far the most common cause of mental incapacity, hence legal incompetence. The legal systems and structures that deal with issues of incapacity have a dual responsibility. Not only are they there to enforce the recognition of the rights of the person with incapacity and protect them from exploitation and abuse, they must also facilitate, not impede, the provision and delivery of needed care and support.

The belief in the absolute right to exercise autonomy is very popular but does not bear intelligent scrutiny. The Law should not allow itself to fail in its responsibility to question the quality of the evidence put before it.

Dementia causes incapacity in several ways that include lack of insight and delusional beliefs amongst other cognitive impairments. I believe that some degree of lack of insight is characteristic of the afflicted. Restiveness to change is natural enough, and life experience may well have made for stoicism, but the refusal of acceptance that assistance in the performance of essential daily activities and therapeutic interventions is necessary is almost universal. Whatever you suggest, the answer tends too often to be 'no'. However, I and any other health practitioner familiar with dementia care can give numerous examples where an intervention, such as attendance at formal day care, had been vigorously resisted, but ultimately became the most enjoyed activity and new routine for the patient, and a valuable form of respite for the life partner.

The right to confidentiality is linked to the issue of capacity. The dogmatic application of this seemingly unconditional right causes great damage and prevents access to vital information when assessments are undertaken. Quite often, the afflicted person's behaviour would in any other context be considered as serious abuse of the partner. The failure to recognise this reveals the inadequacy of the diagnostic and assessment process.

I am guilty and will continue to be technically guilty of providing 'confidential' information to partners, relatives, and key carers of people afflicted with dementia. I do this because I believe that the patient is not the individual, but part of the union, and in providing information to the partner rather than the afflicted person, I am not morally or ethically guilty. My conscience is clear.

There is no clinical encounter without ethical implications. Indeed, ethics, morality, the law, and political ideology are intimately and intricately interwoven. Our beliefs and personal philosophies on these issues determine what we do and how and why we do it.

I will start with a conclusion. Irrespective of who we are and what role we play in the healthcare system, we must always be cognizant of our ethical obligations in the broadest sense. That is the only guarantee that we can give to those who need and use the system that their well-being and best interest is our ultimate goal at all times.

Our medical profession has adhered to a code of ethics for a very long time. To a large degree this is what entitles us doctors to call ourselves a profession. It defines our professionalism and governs our professional behaviour and relationships with our patients, our colleagues and co-workers, our students, and society at large. We are no longer just a self-governing expert association. Our code of ethics is reflected in the Common Law and Acts of Parliament that regulate the shape, scope, and performance of the healthcare system.

Although our code of ethics has ancient origins, it has not stood still; it has had to evolve progressively as society, knowledge, and technology has evolved. It must now incorporate concepts such as human rights and social justice in a very different world than the one in which Hippocrates practised his profession.

Our presumption that everyone unconditionally recognises and respects us as professionals is sadly out of date. There are very few absolutes in life, and acceptance and recognition must be earned, and must continue to be earned. It can be thought of as analogous to Continuing Professional Development, proof of which is now required by our professional organisations and registering bodies.

In common with my whole medical student generation, I was never taught medical ethics. My introduction to the Hippocratic Oath came at an evening meeting that may have been organised by the AMA or the Medical Students Association after we had completed the grinding pre-clinical years of the course and were embarking on our clinical training. This introduction was less than inspirational. One of the honorary surgeons from the Royal Adelaide Hospital read out the Oath between puffs on his cigarette. Nothing of any consequence was presented or discussed, but I managed to irritate him by asking a question, which was testily dismissed. He must have had a more pressing engagement. We would appear to have taken the Oath that ensured that would become ethical practitioners. It was taken for granted that we knew what behaving ethically entailed, and that we would somehow absorb this understanding from observing our teachers, a sort of osmosis by apprenticeship.

A journey of discovery

As soon as I had determined to embark on a career in Geriatric Medicine, I joined the British Geriatrics Society and subscribed to its journal, *Age and Ageing*. I also subscribed to the only other important English language Geriatric journal that I was aware of at the time, the *Journal of the American Geriatric Society* (*JAGS*). *JAGS* was an eye-opener. It was the first and only one among the many professional journals that I read at the time where ethical issues were prominently featured and discussed. The British approach to medical ethics, which we inherited as part of our colonial heritage, differed little from the Australian approach as described above. In America, however, it was taken extremely seriously, and it was not uncommon for very complex ethical issues to be argued in the courts.

The approach in Australia was often what I would describe as 'catechismal'. We had an authoritative list of absolute 'thou shalt not's ...', and a few 'thou shalt do's ...' that could be applied in any given situation without the necessity of troubling the brain. This approach is dangerously simplistic. One sees it to this day, and I will cite numerous examples in the discussion that follows.

Our approach to our ethical obligations is akin to the curate's egg: it is good in parts. We understand that decision-making competence must often be evaluated. Some of us do it very well, many refer it to others because they lack the confidence to do it themselves, and many fail to do it when they should. We have however become quite expert and compliant with the ethical approach to research involving human subjects. Unfortunately, many of us are unaware of the extent of our other ethical obligations and have failed to take them into consideration in our practice.

Very early in my career, I discovered that it was impossible to practise Geriatric Medicine without a deep understanding of medical ethics. As I rose through the ranks and became involved in Palliative Care, and organising and running health services, I made determined efforts to fill this great void in my knowledge and became active in the study of the ethical issues of the day and the application of ethical principles in the delivery of health care. I served on the council of a Bioethics Institute, I wrote position papers, and I made personal submissions to parliamentary inquiries on such issues as euthanasia.

This is the era of the Guideline. However, high-quality guidelines or codes of conduct and medical ethics are in somewhat short supply and are not a discernible part of the numerous practice guidelines that proliferate. I have unearthed two that are current and authoritative. The first is the World Medical Association *Medical Ethics' Manual*. The second is the American *College of Physicians Ethics' Manual*. Both are worthy of study by medical students at any stage of their career.

While these codes of conduct apply equally to all who practise medicine, those of us who have chosen to focus on the health care of the elderly must be constantly aware that we are dealing with a group of people that is almost by definition marginalised and extremely vulnerable. However we define 'elderly', and there are numerous alternatives, we are at risk of creating a social class that is perceived to have common characteristics that go beyond chronological age alone. The very reason that they have been chosen to receive specialised treatment is based on the assumption of health care and other needs arising from degeneration, chronic illness, disability and mental incapacity.

'Individualised' and 'patient-centred care' are terms that have become something of a mantra, but is this what happens in the real world, particularly in long-term care?

Conventional medical ethics

Ethics, morality, the law, and political ideology are intricately interwoven and in essence all rules of conduct or, in a modern context, guidelines, governing our behaviour when forming relationships at every level, from one-on-one relationships, to families, to communities, and to nations. The ultimate purpose of these guidelines is to enable us to live in peace and prosperity and so that individuals can achieve contentment and self-fulfilment and ensure that their progeny can enjoy these same benefits.

In common with most of the modern Western democracies, we hold that the various rules of conduct and laws that are applied in these democracies are secular, and can be arrived at through secular reasoning, irrespective of their historical derivation and development. In other words, there is a necessary and deliberate separation of Church and State. Such are the differences between and within the major religions and the beliefs of numerous minor religions that no religious view can dominate in the modern world with anything close to universal agreement.

Amongst my early readings on bioethics was the very influential textbook *Principles of Biomedical Ethics* by Beauchamp and Childress. It was the first 'primer' that I studied. Although I had read widely, my reading had been somewhat ad hoc and eclectic, related to whatever issue I was pursuing at the time.

Beauchamp and Childress taught that Bioethics is a branch of applied ethics. It represents the application of normative ethical theories, principles and rules to health care provision and practise. They posited that modern bioethics is based on four fundamental and two derived principles:

Fundamental

1. Autonomy (self-determination, the patient's rights)

2. Non-maleficence (do no harm, or at least minimise harm)

3. Beneficence (prevent harm, do good)

4. Justice (give to each his right or due)

Derived

5. Confidentiality

6. Veracity (truth telling)

This approach is known as *Principlism*. This is the perspective that has been so zealously adopted in Australia. I use the word 'perspective' advisedly, as I will explain further. It is only one of several alternative and equally authoritative approaches.

It seems that as a society we need dogma written on tablets of stone that can be applied without the need for thought or deliberation. Dogma and catechisms all derive from some form of higher authority. Principlism meets this need in that its doctrines can be zealously applied without troubling the brain or conscience.

What we accept as the views of deities or founding fathers has to be understood, however, in the context of the time and circumstances in which these commandments, laws and rights were determined and recorded. No one can deny the vile atrocities committed by zealots in the name of a 'Loving God' or charismatic interpreter of totalitarian beliefs.

In my own obsessed and zealous approach to define and understand every concept and term that I am writing about, I read a great deal of philosophical literature. The on-line *Stanford Encyclopedia of Philosophy* became my 'primer'. It did not take very long for me to realise that modern philosophy does not deal in absolutes. There are philosophical views and perspectives on any issue. When seeking definition of specific words and concepts, such as autonomy, rights, principles etc., what one finds in the serious literature is a treatise with no clear conclusion, rather than a simple definition.

Autonomy, relationships, and rights. Who is the patient?

Although the principle of autonomy is only one of four in the above catechism, it has acquired a primacy among the ethical principles. Defining autonomy is as easy as herding cats. Most definitions of it include the concept that it is an individual's capacity for self-determination and/or self-governance, and that our autonomous decisions are rooted in our values and overall commitments and objectives.

Values

There is a lot of talk about 'Australian values'. People are often asked to write down their values so that these will be a guide to substitute decision-making. How many people have ever actually thought about values and all of the possible meanings of the word or concept? Academic literature is full of it. Have you ever tried to define the term? I have. Like all philosophical concepts there are many ways of understanding and defining values. Values can be construed as being ethical, moral, ideological, or social. In most instances, we have not arrived at them by deep thought, we have just picked them up from our parents, our teachers, our clergy and our politicians in a vague and unfocused way because they got us by. They were not seen as particularly important, except in rare moments in our lives that were too uncomfortable to think about until, unfortunately, we experienced them.

In this book, we are examining how we must interact with a person who has a neurodegenerative disease and the resulting manifestations and changes in cognitive function, personality and behaviour. Our patient is not someone with developmental or intellectual disability, or a person with no neuropathology. We are considering mature adults who had 'normal' cognitive capacities and abilities, as well as beliefs and values that were based on their life experience that have become impaired or lost. A critically important part of shaping that experience consists of the relationships that they have had and are currently in.

The Beauchamp and Childress perspective, which has been the main determinant of the conventional understanding, is that the principle of autonomy recognises an individual's right to be self-determining, to make decisions for oneself: 'autonomous actions and choices should not be constrained by others'. It accepts that the person is responsible for his or her own life and has the *right* to make decisions and choices that affect that life. This right is seen as being almost unconditional.

From the outset, this perspective has had, and continues to have, many critics.

Relationships

The main criticism of this perspective centres on the fact that Beauchamp and Childress view the person as an isolated individual, who as of right makes decisions as such an individual. This has been compared to other cultures, particularly Eastern cultures, where the person is seen as a member of family where she is in an interdependent relationship.

In America itself, this has been the stance of eminent feminist philosophers. They have argued that people are socially embedded, and that their identities are formed within the context of social relationships. They argue that the exercise of the right to autonomy must be interpreted in this context.

In the prevailing version of autonomy, we overlook some very basic human attributes. We are social beings, and we have feelings and emotions that we react to and act on. We develop as people within relationships. We need kinship to become who we are and how we behave. At the personal level, we need and strive for deep interpersonal relationships. It defines our personhood.

Maslow's hierarchy of needs is a very compelling summation of human needs (see the chapter on Management) and has played a very significant role in sociological and psychological research. The base of the pyramid is formed by what he called 'deficiency needs'. In order (starting from the base) they are: *Physiological*, *Safety*, *Love and Belonging*, and *Esteem*. The apex of the pyramid is made up by the last need which is *Self-actualisation*.

The commonest and best-known form of a deep interpersonal relationship is marriage, and the debate around same-sex marriage has muddied the waters. Everyone needs such relationships, and people of all races, cultures, personal beliefs and persuasions always have, and always will continue to form them. This is another situation where we must look beyond the trimmings and focus on the gist. The gist is the relationship, irrespective of how it evolved and who sanctions and recognises it.

Relationship is also a very well-studied subject. However two people meet and decide to form a relationship, it evolves and develops (as Erikson's theory suggests). Ultimately there is a mutual commitment that requires trust. A healthy and successful attachment provides a sense of safety and security and facilitates effective functioning. Decisions in all domains, roles and responsibilities are shared. In the context of the relationship we stop being highly self-centred and individualistic, and merge into an interdependent partnership.

Human beings have emotions and feelings that determine our perceptions and our actions. The cement in our deepest relationships is love. This too is a well-studied topic. The perspective that most closely defines the conclusions that I have reached intuitively is 'Love as Union'. The result is that lovers come to share the interests, roles, virtues, and so on, that constitute what formerly was two individual identities, but now has become a shared identity, and they do so in part by each allowing the other to play an important role in defining his own identity.

The word 'marriage' has become an obstacle to rational debate, and the term tends to be associated particularly with the legal rights linked with this type of relationship. I would suggest that it should be replaced by the word 'Union', although I am not hopeful that our society has evolved enough rational maturity to make this possible.

My evidence base is built from the experience of getting to know thousands of patients, partners, and relatives in their darkest moments, when confronted with the possibility that one of them is afflicted by dementia.

The wife of one of my patients put it succinctly. She was severely disabled with rheumatoid arthritis, and he had moderately severe dementia. She told me that they had been married for 60 years, and progressively she had become the brains of the family, while he was the legs. They both continued to love and need each other, but increasing difficulty was arising due to emerging behavioural problems and his increasing cognitive impairment. She wanted help and advice to enable her to continue coping in order to sustain the relationship.

I have now seen many, many patients presenting with quite advanced dementia after the death of a spouse. Often, nothing had been suspected by close relatives and friends until that time. That social unit, that partnership, continued to function because the healthy partner took on new roles and responsibilities and supported the other partner in continuing in a meaningful and valued role. In these situations, the surviving partner often had sufficient social skills which had sustained her public image, her social façade alongside her husband.

When both partners are alive, the relationship is a huge part of the patient's coping capacity. In earlier times and in more primitive societies, the afflicted one's very life depended on the partner. Dementia threatens and damages that relationship.

This relationship is the most important thing in the patient's life. I have seen many patients with dementia suffering from depression. I explore their feelings and sense of hopelessness. I have seen many patients who believed that their life is no longer worth living and that they be better off dead, but vigorously denied suicidal thoughts and intent saying, 'I could never do that to my husband ... To my family.'

In my experience, separation anxiety, the sheer terror that the life partner will abandon, or already has abandoned, the afflicted partner is quite common, and not just in the late stages of dementia. I believe that it is greatly underestimated and underdiagnosed in the literature. As I explain in detail further in the book, I almost always interview and examine the patient alone first; I then interview the life partner, relative or key carer privately. It is the partner, not the patient, who *perceives and experiences the impact* of separation anxiety. If the assessor does not do this (as is the current norm), many vitally important issues will not be recognised.

That union persists until death. I regularly see patients with very advanced dementia who cannot remember that they are married and who the partner is, yet somehow they sense the presence of that person and respond to that presence in the way that they do not respond to anybody else. I tell partners and relatives that this is my belief, and they are comforted by it.

I believe that forming relationships is a biological imperative. To survive, a species must reproduce and ensure the survival of its progeny. Many species mate for life, ensuring that they not only reproduce but remain together to nurture their young. There is strength in numbers, and successful species form groups: herds, prides, gaggles, et cetera, et cetera. There is strength and harmony within the group.

The development of the neocortex gave humanity the capacity to develop complex societies that led to the great civilisations we see today. This was only possible because of the human capacity to coexist peacefully and cooperatively in individual and large group relationships. These capacities include all of the things that I list among the 'Frontal Lobe' behavioural and personality changes: insight, empathy, compassion, impulse control, and emotional stability. These are underdeveloped in ADHD; they are never developed in some personality disorders; and they are damaged in dementia.

Autonomy is accepted as a human right. I believe that the right to make relationships is based on a more fundamental human need and should be recognised and promoted with equal zeal.

In the context of dementia, the concept of relationship cannot be overstated. For the patient, there is a hierarchy of relationships. The key one is the relationship with the life partner. Then there are close family members and friends who can step into that breach when the life partner is no longer there. Thereafter, anyone who deals with the patient in any way must first form a relationship of trust. All skilled aged care workers understand this.

As doctors, we must enter into such a relationship, as must nurses and other caregivers. The quality of these relationships will determine how successful any supportive and therapeutic interventions will be.

When I think and talk about the importance of relationships almost everyone I know and meet believes that this is self-evident.

Who is the patient?

When I returned to Australia as a geriatrician in the early 1970s, I was faced with the task of creating a niche for this new specialty among the specialties already in place. Geriatricians were seen as a particular threat to General Physicians. In my writings and presentations, including one at a College of Physicians Annual Scientific Meeting, I put forward the concept that one of the key differences between Geriatricians and General Physicians was that we focused on the 'Family Unit', not just the individual patient.

In dementia, and in virtually every other chronic disease, there is no single owner of the problem. It affects the whole relationship. In more recent times I have taken to using the term *life partner* as it is more personal, clearer and warmer than 'social/family unit' and does not require the form of the relationship to dominate our thinking.

I truly believe this, and I have openly put this belief into my practice of geriatric medicine for close to half a century.

Several prominent authors have emphasised the importance of understanding the role and the needs of *carers* of the person with dementia. This is almost my message, but they do not go far enough. They continue to describe the carers as someone who is outside or alongside the person with dementia, but not intrinsically *a participant* in the dementing process.

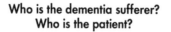

Who is the dementia sufferer?
Who is the patient?

He has dementia

She has a problem

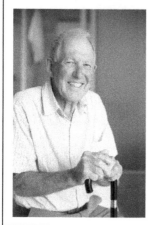
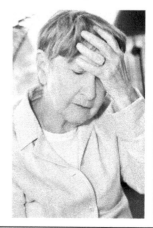

When an elderly couple presents to the GP, and one of them has pneumonia, there is no question of who the patient is. The afflicted one has all the symptoms and does all of the suffering. That is what the medical model is all about. This is the patient with whom we form a doctor/patient relationship. That is right and proper *in this context*.

When an elderly couple presents to the GP because the husband has dementia complicated by paranoid thinking and aggressive behaviour, which he does not recognise nor accept as true, who then is the patient? He has no complaints, there is 'nothing wrong with ~~him~~ me', and he needs nothing. She is the only one in this situation who is actually suffering, and her suffering is often very severe. It would not be there if he was not afflicted. Can the consultation or any resulting intervention then be solely directed at him?

The question 'Whose problem is it?' has always served me well when approaching complex and difficult situations.

In the context of dementia, the patient is not an individual. The 'patient' is a union, a composite, a dyad, a life-partnership comprised of two people, who are inextricably inter-dependent, and each significantly affected by the disease in different ways. The needs of both must be equally understood and simultaneously addressed.

This is not a revolutionary concept. There is a very relevant precedent in Couple and Family Therapy. It is recognised as a legitimate sub-specialty in Psychiatry. A textbook and manuals are available under the banner of the American Psychiatric Association. Last year, the American Association for Marriage and Family Therapy published a Code of Ethics that differs very little from similar codes published by Medical, Nursing and Allied Health Professional organisations.

It is interesting to observe that I have presented my views to a variety of audiences on different occasions many, many times. When speaking at formal meetings with people from medical specialties and aged care organisations, my views are seen as heretical by many. When I have discussed these views with audiences largely comprising of nurses, social workers or carers, they have been lauded as being 'spot on'.

I deliberately and routinely interview the patient and the partner separately. Proponents of the absolute right to autonomy usually include the right of the elderly 'clients' to have 'an advocate of their choice' when faced with a clinical consultation or assessment. This exposes the underlying assumption that elderly people are part of a class that may not be capable of resisting the grasp for power by the clinician. This is discrimination and the extreme opposite of the recognition of autonomy.

Another criticism of the application of the perspective of autonomy is that it is coldly academic and legalistic. The failure to consider the person in the context of a relationship is also a failure to recognise the impact that feelings play in shaping beliefs and influencing decision-making.

The person with moderate to advanced dementia is often very conflicted. Many of these patients regularly thank me for the opportunity to see me alone because they have grievances against the life partner that they want to divulge. They feel unfairly judged, since there is nothing wrong with them, but things are being done as if there was. They are always being criticised and told what to do. The partner is conspiring with the family to put them in a nursing home or take away their driver's licence. No one listens to them.

They are more open with these criticisms than with admissions of their total emotional dependence on that same person. I have seen instances when the partner has been accused of elder abuse because of such complaints being voiced to agency aged care workers, and many more accusations that the partner is not honouring the patient's right to autonomy.

Those who subscribe to this version of what constitutes autonomy are seen as benevolent and politically correct. After all, this version is written into legislation, such as the Advanced Care Directives Act, South Australia 2013, and enforced by law.

Those who question this interpretation and its application are perceived as asserting their power over someone who is powerless, for their own selfish purposes.

Services that purport to respect the right to autonomy and call themselves consumer-driven, or even better, client-centred and client-directed, can almost be assured of government approbation and funding. I must stress that I am not criticising or belittling these concepts, but making the point that these words, like the word 'autonomy' itself, have acquired an aura of instant rightness, acceptance and credibility. We question these words, and bring attention to the harm that this approach may cause, at our peril. This has led me to coin a term, 'Benevolent Ageism'.

Needs, wants and rights

There is a tendency to claim that all wants are needs and that this makes them 'rights'.

Need is frequently referred to, but it is seldom defined, on the assumption that it is a self-evident concept.

Bradshaw (1977) offered a useful taxonomy that has helped me to understand the concept. He defined four categories of need. The first was *normative need*, i.e. need that has been defined by experts in a given field as representing need in a particular situation or context. It requires the establishment of objectives and desired standards and is in part a reflection of the community's aspirations in health and social welfare. Anyone falling short of the desired standard is considered to be in need.

The second is *felt need* or *want*. By itself, it is an inadequate measure of real need, being limited by the individual's perceptions and knowledge of alternative options. Want can of course be present in the absence of normative need.

The third is *expressed need*, or *demand*. This is felt need put into action. It still depends on the individual's perceptions and knowledge of alternatives.

The final variety of need is *comparative need*. This is determined by studying the characteristics of people in receipt of a service and by extrapolation defining all those who have similar characteristics, but do not receive the service, as being in need. This can be used in planning to identify 'at risk' populations and to set numerical service provision guidelines.

The unconditional right to autonomy. Consequences matter

The conventional version of autonomy poses a threat to the delivery of needed care, as the client may be given the choice of the fulfilment of a want rather than an assessed need, which will often be a cheaper alternative for the funder: 'I don't want you to dress my ulcer today, I'd rather have an hour's worth of gardening'. (This was an actual example given at the launch of 'My Aged Care' at a country town.)

The derived principles of confidentiality and veracity are strongly linked to the prevailing perspective of autonomy, and hence impact on the proposition that the patient is a union with another or others.

It is easy to understand that confidentiality protects the one-to-one interaction between the patient and the practitioner. The geriatric situation is, however, frequently much more complicated than any typical consultation, as it involves team members, other practitioners and agencies, as well as partners, relatives and carers. There are also clinical records, which may be accessed by a variety of clinicians and non-clinical workers. In general, only the practitioner's obligation to the law overrides the patient's right to confidentiality.

The most troubling issue is that in practice, in everyday life, the life partner or key carer is regularly excluded from access to information that affects the whole relationship.

It is not at all rare that the 'informal' caregiver, who is denied critical care information, is subsequently legally appointed as the formal Guardian and obligatory recipient of all of the same information that she was ineligible to receive the day before.

I interpret 'veracity' and the 'right to know' in similar ways. I have many colleagues who conclude their assessment with such information as, 'You have got mild Alzheimer's Disease'. They are blissfully unaware of the harm that they are doing. This is maleficence. Information can harm. What, when and how we convey information to our patient requires careful consideration.

People with cognitive impairment are anxious and dread hearing these words. For many of them this is tantamount to the declaration of the end of their life as they know it. They fear that this will inevitably result in admission to a nursing home with a loss of all the relationships and liberties that they treasure.

I regularly see people who are hurt and enraged by the conclusions of assessments and tribunal hearings. They are not informed. They do not have the capacity to understand the decisions in any other way. Their suspicions are confirmed, and someone, the partner and the referring doctor, pays the price.

When difficult decisions, such as the cancellation of a driver's license, have to be made I make sure that neither the partner nor the GP is seen as culpable and that I bear the blame. I am the bad cop, the relationship with the GP is much more important than the relationship with me.

In the separate interview that I have with the partner, I conclude with a detailed and honest explanation of the process and implications of dementia. I offer counselling and a care plan. The ethical obligation is met, because the true patient, the union, now has the necessary information to manage the issues. Information can harm if the receiver of that information does not have the capacity to understand it and deal with its implications.

The anecdote above raises critically important issues about how the current interpretation of confidentiality creates barriers to the acquisition of information that is needed to provide necessary support to people afflicted with dementia. It has become very difficult to obtain information on the findings of assessments conducted by government-appointed assessment teams and individuals. When I am undertaking an assessment on referral from a patient's general practitioner, and I try to access all the relevant information, I regularly find it impossible to obtain that information. This is not just something that happens in South Australia. I have been involved in a number of cases interstate, and I have found the same problems.

Mental capacity and competence

Issues related to competence and/or capacity are the most frequent ethical concerns in gerontological practice. In our usage, the word 'competence' is a legal concept. What the clinician has to establish is 'capacity'. These terms are often used interchangeably, and the opposite applies in the British and the American literature.

Although there is a widespread belief that autonomy is an unconditional right, no right can be unconditional. The autonomous action must be morally, legally and, at times, socially acceptable. The limits of autonomy are determined by society and the law.

I would remind the reader of the definition of autonomy discussed above. An autonomous agent must have the ability to govern herself when she acts, to rationally reflect upon and evaluate her reasoning in reaching a decision, and to discern consequences. This is what has to be demonstrated when capacity is being questioned.

Mental incapacity was defined in the South Australian *Guardianship and Administration Act, 1993* as:

… the inability of a person to look after his or her own health, safety or welfare or to manage his or her own affairs, as a result of

(a) any damage to, or any illness, disorder, imperfect or delayed development, impairment or deterioration, of the brain or mind; or

(b) any physical illness or condition that renders the person incapable to communicate his or her intentions or wishes in any manner whatsoever.

The causes of mental incapacity can include dementia, intellectual disability, brain damage, mental illness, coma or being in a moribund state.

The South Australian *Advanced Care Directives Act 2013* replaced or amended a number of pre-existing and related Acts, including the *Consent to Medical Treatment and Palliative Care Act 1995*, *Coroners Act 2003*, *Fair Work Act 1994* and *Guardianship and Administration Act 1993*.

This resulted in all decisions being treated as serious health care, 'life and death' decisions. In dementia, however, most of the decisions under consideration are not of this ilk. They are day-to-day decisions that may seem trivial to the uninformed observer who is unaware of their importance in the context. In other words, we generalise from the dramatic to the seemingly mundane.

This has resulted in a sort of hierarchy of decisions and the division of Guardianship into the categories of 'Lifestyle' and 'Medical'. The most superficial analysis shows that this is nonsensical, and counter to the whole concept of the bio-psycho-social perspective of the causation of illness.

The above Act defines impaired decision-making capacity in terms of the capability of understanding information relevant to the decision in question, including consequences; retaining such information; using the information in the course of making the decision; and communicating that decision. This is a fairly conventional list:

> (1) For the purposes of this Act, a person will be taken to have impaired decision-making capacity in respect of a particular decision if –
>
> (a) the person is not capable of –
>
>> (i) understanding any information that may be relevant to the decision (including information relating to the consequences of making a particular decision); or
>>
>> (ii) retaining such information; or

(iii) using such information in the course of making the decision; or

(iv) communicating his or her decision in any manner; or

(b) the person has satisfied any requirement in an advance care directive given by the person that sets out when he or she is to be considered to have impaired decision-making capacity (however described) in respect of a decision of the relevant kind.

(2) For the purposes of this Act –

(a) a person will not be taken to be incapable of understanding information merely because the person is not able to understand matters of a technical or trivial nature; and

(b) a person will not be taken to be incapable of retaining information merely because the person can only retain the information for a limited time; and

(c) a person may fluctuate between having impaired decision-making capacity and full decision-making capacity; and

(d) a person's decision-making capacity will

not be taken to be impaired merely because a
decision made by the person results, or may
result, in an adverse outcome for the person.

As in the *Guardianship and Administration Act 1993*,
the definitions of capacity are often accompanied by a list
of conditions that may cause incapacity.

These rules, guidelines, call them what you will, were
developed when neuroscience, including neuropsychology,
was in its infancy. Psychologists, neuropsychologists, and
other neuroscientists have studied each of these factors,
these capabilities, and have taken them far beyond the
realms of academic philosophical speculation. Processes
such as reasoning, comprehension and judgement are no
longer abstract, but are grounded in solid neurophysiological
evidence.

It is also no longer accepted that people with certain
diagnoses, such as Alzheimer's disease, are automatically
deemed globally incapable of making decisions.

The process

Those of us who are required to determine capacity or
capability should not only be aware of the causes (the
pathological diagnosis), but also the cognitive functions
and behavioural attributes that lead to the loss or

impairment of any of these capabilities (see below).

When asked to determine the capacity of any patient, I treat this like a new case-taking in accordance with my practice protocol, and I interview the patient and life partner, carer or relative separately in my usual way. If further corroborating evidence is required I approach relevant sources with the consent of the patient or through the briefing solicitor.

My personal focus always remains on what I perceive to be the patient's (as defined above) best interest, irrespective of who may wish to influence or question my decision.

The following discussion deals with the formal evaluation of capacity, but in every clinical encounter where the cognitive state is of concern, we of necessity also make *informal* evaluations. We have to make judgements about the patient's ability to engage, to communicate, memory, mood, thinking, and so on. By the end of an interview we have a reasonable assessment of the patient's mental capacity. We have to do this in order to make appropriate care-planning decisions. It takes little additional effort to formalise the process.

There is a commonly held belief that the question someone is capacity to make decisions is an offence against the right to autonomy, and assessment should only be undertaken when there is an important decision in the offing. What makes a decision important is *the context and the consequences.* It is not just such hefty decisions as whether or not to undergo a mastectomy or to sell the house. Failure to adhere to strict daily routines can become an intolerable burden for the partner and result in the breakdown of care at home. Can this person make a rapid and appropriate decision in the event of a crisis while driving?

It must always be remembered that dementia is about change. *This is a critical contextual point.* We need to understand the patient's history. Would this person be exercising her 'right' to make this particular decision, which will cause hardship and concern for her life-partner, or expose her to risk that is counter to her best interest, if we were seeing her before the emergence of the manifestations of dementia?

Assessing capabilities, competence, and capacity

In the context of a decision having to be made, *competence* involves several capabilities, including the capacity to:

1. Understand the facts involved in the decision and of the options available.

2. Appreciate the nature and significance of the decision being faced.

3. Integrate and order information and consequences of acting (or not acting) on

the various options (reasoning).

4. Select an option and give cogent reasons.

5. Evaluate risks and benefits in terms of personal values (appreciation).

6. Persevere in the choice of options (consistency).

Thus, the decision-making should reflect consistency, rationality, awareness of influencing factors, in the context of cultural and social issues. And there are two elements to such decision-making capacity, *a cognitive element*, knowing and understanding; and *a functional element*, being able to undertake the activities required to achieve an outcome. Both of these elements should be clinically analysed.

To begin with, we must have perception and insight in order to have a realistic and current understanding of our circumstances, and the context within which the decision is to be made. We must also have a realistic perception of our capabilities and disabilities to put the decision into effect. We must have the ability to reason and to understand the consequences of alternative future scenarios.

Insight and executive function are central to realistic, effective, and capable decision-making.

The significance of insight

It is generally understood that the loss of insight, the awareness of change, is a well-recognised manifestation in all forms of dementia. In its most extreme form it is labelled *anosognosia*, the complete inability to perceive that there is a major impairment. The significance of the loss of insight is however greatly underestimated. It is something that passing reference is made to during a consultation, but its presence and severity is rarely specifically looked for. I strongly commend the book *Insight in Psychiatry* by Ivana S Markova[*] as obligatory reading.

Because of the way that I undertake an assessment I have become increasingly convinced that lack of insight is common even in early dementia. I ask each patient why they were referred to see me. The majority with mild to moderate dementia do not understand that they have been referred for a cognitive assessment. Many of those who are aware of this, preface it by explaining that their partner or relative has questioned their memory, and they have agreed to the assessment even though they do not believe it to be necessary. Even those who complain of failing memory at the outset, deny or minimise memory loss when directly addressed.

They are not aware of the cognitive impairment and its consequences. The patient is not lying (as one GP

[*]   Marková, I. (2005). *Insight in Psychiatry*. Cambridge: Cambridge University Press. doi:10.1017/CBO9780511543999

indignantly insisted), it is a neurologically-based inability to perceive the reality in the same way as those around her. I believe that it is a largely failure of executive function. It is a cause of incapacity that is often missed or dismissed because overall the dementia may not seem to be severe enough to raise questions about capacity and competence. The common practice of interviewing only the patient and not interviewing the life-partner/carer separately means that glaring examples of lack of insight are regularly missed.

I commonly see patients who cause great concern for their families and carers because of their cognitive decline. At the interview, a significant proportion of these patients will rate themselves as completely capable in all of the basic and instrumental activities of daily living and will say that they actually perform all of these activities independently. They cannot understand the concern of those around them, because *from their perspective* there is no problem, and no need for any kind of assistance or intervention. They can sound quite convincing, but if the relative is interviewed privately, as is my almost invariable practice, the reality that is revealed is quite contrary to the patient's perception: 'mother has not cooked for years … I do the shopping … She never leaves the house … I do the washing, she can't use her washing machine … She insists that she showers herself, but she is incontinent and she smells …'

If we are primed by a dogmatic belief in 'the right to autonomy' and the associated beliefs in what constitutes confidentiality, we are quite likely to miss this diagnosis. It is easy to miss and unfortunately a great many general practitioners, neurologists, psychiatrists, and, alas, geriatricians do miss it. This, and the reliance on simple screening tests as absolute evidence for or against the presence of a cognitive impairment and measures of severity, is a failure of due process.

The primacy of executive function

The focus on memory and measures of memory as the definitive cognitive failure in dementia has led to an inability to recognise that it is the loss of the executive function that is the most damaging loss. You can have all the memories in the world, but they are of no use if you cannot use them in a meaningful way.

Executive function, which controls and coordinates virtually all of our cognitive processes, as well as integrating all other relevant sensory inputs and motor functions involved in even the simplest action, is the most significant loss in dementia. Executive function is what enables us to make reasonable judgements and to take the probable consequences of an action into account. This ability is one of the key criteria for determining capacity.

Changes in personality and behaviour

In addition to these cognitive impairments, people afflicted with dementia often develop changes in personality and behaviour that I group simply as the result of frontal lobe damage. These include a lack of inhibition, impulsivity, a loss of empathy and compassion, and impaired capacity to cope with personal relationships. The impact on valid and rational decision-making capacity should be obvious. I continue to remind the reader that we are talking about change, and that the decisions and behaviours in question would have been very different when this same person was in full possession of her powers.

Autonomy and independence

Lay people, the partners, relatives and carers of the people afflicted with dementia, tend to equate autonomy with independence, to independent functioning. I frequently hear such remarks has, 'I try not to help mum too much because I don't want to rob her of her independence'. Another common one is, 'If you take away dad's licence, you will take away his independence'.

For a long time, we have measured independence in terms of the capability to perform *the basic and instrumental activities of daily living*. Whether we realise it or not, performance is a very practical way to measure executive function. Indeed, several Occupational Therapy instruments are designed do just that. When we compare the afflicted person's apparent perception of the capability with the observations of the actual performance by the partner (in separate private interviews), we have strong evidence of any loss of insight and of any loss of executive function.

Our conclusions should always be accompanied by this kind of evidence. When we fail to do this, the presumption that capacity/capability exists unless proven otherwise pertains. The harm that then results to the afflicted person or partner from actions taken by the supposedly autonomous afflicted person is a failure of the assessor, and where a legal examination has taken place, of the legal examiner for not insisting on the production of relevant evidence or accepting poor quality evidence at face value. I deal with this in greater detail in the chapter on the Initial Assessment.

Practical examples

As observed above, the elderly patient has generally been competent in the past, and specific situations arise that make it necessary to test the *retention* of that competence. In some instances, as in severe dementia, there may almost be a general incompetence to make decisions across the whole spectrum of decision making. More commonly, there is limited incompetence, with the inability to make some complex decisions, but the capacity to make decisions on simpler, more clear-cut issues (with the reservations discussed above). Two contextual examples are given below.

Elements of assessment in issues involving property and finance

In determining if the person has the capacity to make a decision, the assessor must determine if, in relation to the issue at hand, the person:

- Knows and understands his/her
  - assets and income
  - debts and expenses
  - obligations, such as paying bills on time, and obligations to the family and others

- Has the ability to
  - budget as necessary (to balance the budget)
  - perform necessary calculations
  - weigh the risks and benefits and appreciate the consequences of a course of action

- detect and avoid fraud and exploitation

Testamentary capacity

The test for testamentary capacity is a common law test, classically stated in the 1870 United Kingdom case of *Banks v Goodfellow*. This remains the advice given to doctors by lawyers to this day.

According to *Banks v Goodfellow*, in order to have the requisite soundness of mind the person must:

1. understand the nature and effect of a will;

2. understand the nature and extent of their property;

3. comprehend and appreciate the claims to which they ought to give effect;

4. be suffering from no disorder of the mind or insane delusion that would result in an unwanted disposition.

Proper evaluation of capacity in these situations is very dependent on the availability of corroborating information, which is at times very difficult to obtain, particularly where the principal informant has an obvious conflict of interest.

Consent

A valid consent must satisfy the following conditions

1. It must be freely and voluntarily given;

2. It must cover the procedure (or course of action) to be medically performed;

3. It must cover the person who is to perform the medical procedure;

4. It must be given by a patient who is competent, and what time do we have to be there right;

5. It must be informed.

Who can consent on behalf of the patient?

Legislation governing decisions about competence tends to view all decision-making in terms of consent to medical procedures. As an example, in South Australia, the *Advance Care Directives Act 2013* has replaced Enduring Power Of Guardianship, Medical Power Of Attorney and anticipatory directions documents which had been very specific. As discussed, this has resulted in a hierarchy of decisions that devalues and trivialises other decisions.

Much, much more often in the context of dementia, however, the decisions that need to be made are in the realms of 'lifestyle' rather than medical matters. They are everyday decisions about the basic and instrumental activities of daily living, safety, welfare and social conduct. It must be remembered that these are decisions that are made several times every day. Many of these lifestyle decisions are deemed to be trivial and unimportant. Some of the lifestyle decisions seem so obviously benign that capacity requires no consideration; such decisions as when to go to bed, when to have a meal, not to have a shower.

This separation of decisions between important and unimportant, reflects the lack of understanding of dementia by those who drafted the legislation and their advisors. They have not understood the significance of loss of insight, and how difficult it is for the life partner or the carer to establish routines that make life tolerable. These 'trivial' decisions can have a very significant impact on the patient's safety, care, and well-being, and may cause concern, great difficulty, and distress to the life-partner (the other half of the union).

I recall one situation where I persuaded a very stressed and nearly exhausted partner to avail herself of an offer of a respite admission for her husband. When I next met her after his return home, she told me angrily, 'If that is what respite is, you can keep it'. While he was a resident at the aged care facility he was able to decide when to go to bed, when to get up, to refuse to shower, and even to resume smoking (in an outside area dedicated for this purpose).

The proud philosophy of the organisation was total respect for the person's autonomy. She had to painfully re-establish all the routines that had enabled her to survive and keep him at home with her and viewed all further offers of outside assistance with suspicion. I could give many similar examples in home care.

This kind of all-purpose legislation can also put restrictions on who can be the substitute decision-maker, when the most obvious and appropriate decision-maker is someone who has a deep personal relationship with that person. In some situations, if the life partner is a doctor or a nurse they may be deemed inappropriate substitute decision-makers because of a conceivable (bizarre) conflict of interest in critical situations.

The principles of substitute decision-making:

The substitute decision-maker should be guided by the following principles:

- what the wishes of the person would have been if he or she had not become mentally incapacitated (where this can be determined);

- the present wishes of the person, if these can be expressed;

- whether or not existing informal arrangements for the treatment and care of the person are adequate (if so, these should not be disturbed);

- which decision or legal order would be least restrictive of the person's rights and personal autonomy, whilst still ensuring his or her proper care and protection.

In reality, the substitute decision-maker has to become a quasi-case manager. In my experience, legally-appointed guardians, who are not relatives or friends, tend to see their role as zealously defending the clients right to autonomy, rather than making care decisions, and monitoring consequences. The differentiation between 'medical' and 'lifestyle' care decisions is spelt out in relevant legislation in some of the various States.

Paternalism

Professional caregivers, particularly medical practitioners and nurses, are often accused of paternalism, or the more politically correct 'parentalism', which is deemed by the critic to be a deliberate failure of recognition of the patient's right to autonomy.

The *South Australian Aged Care Directives Act 2013*

contains the following clause:

> 7-(2) (d) a person's decisionmaking capacity will
> not be taken to be impaired merely because a
> decision made by the person results, or may result,
> in an adverse outcome for the person.

This is of course intended to apply to people who otherwise meet all the criteria to be deemed to have capacity, but as I have argued above, there are many very vulnerable people who are presumed to have capacity because causes of incapacity (other than the pathological diagnosis) have not been properly identified.

In the context of dementia, probably the commonest exercise of 'autonomy' that I see is refusal of needed services. The rationalisation put forward is often along the lines of, 'she wants control'; 'she wants to preserve her independence'; 'she doesn't want strangers coming into her home'; and other platitudes that reflect the observer's inability to 'get inside the patient's head' and realise that she has no understanding of her situation and its implications.

'Keeping people home at all costs' is an idealised objective of aged care. It is certainly what almost every patient will tell you that they want. It is associated with a lack of insight and resistance to change that is almost universal in dementia. The question that generally remains unanswered is, what is the cost, and who pays it? While the financial cost may be great, the emotional cost paid by the life partner is often greater. It is not a pile of bricks that matters. As they say in the classics, 'home is where the heart is'; it is the relationship that the patient wants to preserve at all costs.

In making rulings that enforce this 'right', the Law is often acting on very poor and inadequate evidence. This is not the fault of the Law, but of the authors of the legislation, and the practitioners who fail to recognise the evidence of incapacity, which alas includes many of us.

The terms 'patient-centred', 'client-centred', 'patient-directed', etcetera, are coming to be included in every program, guideline and policy. It is the new orthodoxy and mantra. I must confess that I am somewhat bemused, because I regularly see examples of very bad practice that have deleterious outcomes for those who we are trying to treat and assist under this rubric. I believe that in adhering to my ethical principles what I do is completely patient-centred, and I explain this to the patient, the life-partner and any involved relatives.

Choosing between therapeutic options has significant limits, determined by the patient's insight, comprehension and knowledge. When I have consulted my cardiologists, I have accepted that they have a far greater knowledge and understanding of the options that I have and that at times there are no feasible alternatives. I have a pacemaker. Although I signed a consent that listed all the conceivable complications, refusal was never going be this patient's choice. Can the average patient distinguish one antidepressant from another, or the optimal anti-hypertensive cocktail rather than mono-therapy?

It is right and proper that all decisions to intervene in any way are supported by an explanation and why that alternative was chosen in comprehensible terms, but if the patient or someone on behalf of a patient demands an alternative that I believe is contrary to the patient's best interest, despite my explanation, I withdraw from the situation and suggest that they find an alternative opinion.

It is interesting to observe that many partners and relatives go straight to Google following a consultation with the patient's GP. They look up each medication and focus on the adverse effects. They then question the practitioner's choices and approaches to management, sometimes very aggressively. I frequently have to explain that the lists of adverse effects are first compiled during drug trials and the tables show comparisons between the active agent and the placebo taken by the control group. Not all of the listed Adverse Drug Reactions (ADRs) are necessarily caused by the medication and some are exceedingly rare. Some are even found in the placebo group more often in the treatment group. I try not to be a prescriber, but I always discuss what I will be recommending in detail to the GP, and we go through a Risk/Benefit analysis in the context of the patient's situation, which is often palliative/the end of life. I generally, but not always succeed.

It is important to understand that technical information in any field needs to be interpreted and explained by someone who understands it. The obvious person, who meets the criteria is the General Practitioner.

Non-maleficence & beneficence

I will deal with these two principles together, as each has been nominated as the most important principle by important philosophers, and as I believe they are both sides of the same coin. It could be argued that they seek an almost identical end.

Healthcare professionals have a duty of care. While respect for autonomy may be one of the principles that are the foundation of medical ethics, but so also are non-maleficence and beneficence principles that underlie how we carry out our duties, and how we will be judged if we fail in this responsibility.

When we are part of a Geriatric or Psychogeriatric Service that duty of care applies to all situations, including Residential Care.

I can rightly claim that by my actions I regularly

restore capacity, hence autonomy, to someone who had lost it temporarily – as can any health professional, by treating conditions that result in loss of capacity.

The term *beneficence* connotes all forms of action intended to benefit or promote the good of other persons. It is seen as a moral obligation to act for the benefit of our patients by helping them to further their important and legitimate interests, often by preventing or removing possible harms.

In this, the needs and interests of the patient take precedence over other concerns. While we must be conscious of our responsibility to society, or the institution in which we work, once we have entered into a doctor–patient relationship we must give primacy to the patient. This assumes, of course, that we are dealing with conventional interventions that would be generally available in a given society. Our duty of care comes under this rubric. Of course, by patient in this context I mean the union, the partnership.

Beneficence can at times also be construed as paternalism, when the practitioner acts in what he construes to be the best interests of the patient without consideration of the patient's viewpoint, or even against the patient's stated wishes, on the grounds that the practitioner has superior knowledge. This generally involves making practical assumptions about the patient's capacity to make decisions, or to handle information and disclosure, without a formal assessment of capacity.

I find that patients and families accept my assurance that my sole concern is the well-being of the patient, irrespective of anyone else's viewpoint or any pressure being exerted by any agency, particularly a hospital, and that I will act as the patient's advocate to ensure access to any resource that is available. Many patients with dementia need this to be explicitly stated at the outset of a consultation.

Very prominent philosophers such as Immanuel Kant and David Hume considered beneficence to be the prime moral principle.

The principle of non-maleficence is often stated as 'Above all, do no harm' (*Primum non nocere*). The Hippocratic Oath includes the statement: 'I will use treatment to help the sick according to my ability and judgement, but I will never use it to injure or wrong them.' Many authorities consider non-maleficence, rather than beneficence or autonomy, as the overriding bioethical principle.

Harm can be defined as 'physical or mental damage; mischief, hurt, disservice; a material or tangible detriment or loss to a person' (Webster's Dictionary). Much of what is done in the name of autonomy could meet this definition.

As the practitioner owes the patient a duty of care, his or her actions must reflect *due care*. This requires that the practitioner demonstrates specialised knowledge, skill, competence and diligence in their dealings with patients.

These attributes are measured against the standards expected of 'an ordinary and competent practitioner'. In the case of the aged, the practitioner must be very aware of the particular vulnerability of the patient.

Good communication is central to good/due care. Much of the dissatisfaction with health care in all situations stems from poor communication rather than poor practice.

One attribute of due care is the appropriate referral of patients to those with higher order skills in the management of a particular disorder. Some general practitioners are reluctant to refer patients with dementia for specialist opinion, because they believe that nothing can be done, for the reason that they think only in terms of prescription and have no faith in the efficacy of available medication.

End of life decisions

The issue of euthanasia is frequently discussed. The concept enjoys a high degree of popular support and the right to choose the manner of one's dying is again seen as unconditional by many people.

In the context of terminal illness there are a number of ethical considerations. We must:

1. advance the patient's well-being by offering freedom from physical, emotional, and

spiritual distress by appropriate therapy and intervention;

2. provide all necessary information to enable the patient or the patient's proxy to make informed choices;

3. accept the competent patient's right to accept or reject any medical care recommended;

4. ascertain and recognise the patient's wishes about the initiation, continuation, or cessation of life-sustaining treatment;

5. inform the patient when your personal morality would influence the recommendation or practice of any medical procedure that the patient needs or wants.

There are both moral and legal deterrents to the taking of human life. The argument for euthanasia appeals to the principle of autonomy – that the competent person should be allowed to make decisions about such issues as accepting medical interventions, including life-supporting or sustaining interventions, and determining at which point life is no longer acceptable. As always, the greatest dilemmas arise in the context of diminished capacity.

In the advanced, palliative phase for the patient we must focus on the relief and prevention of all forms of distress, comfort, safety, and the promotion of the highest quality of life that can be managed in the circumstances. We must also support and succour those who have a deep abiding personal relationship with that patient and who are undergoing the same trauma.

There are ways of ensuring that the wishes of the patient are honoured beyond the point of incompetence. These include Living Wills, Advance Directives and the legal granting of Enduring Powers for substitute decision-making.

Justice

Justice is not a simple concept. Most would accept that we should act fairly, without selective favour on the basis of wealth, sex, age, religion or race. In reality, when resources are scarce, society tends to give preference to the young, at the expense of the aged. The wealthy can generally access any service that they need, when the poor cannot. They can also exert political influence to determine how scarce resources are distributed.

The key point used to characterise a just stance is a belief that similar individuals should have equal consideration of their interests, equal opportunity to further those interests, equal access to society's institutions, and an equitable share of society's resources.

I believe that as a society, as a profession, many of us as individuals are guilty of failing to deal justly with our patients. We discriminate against the aged. There is a tacit acceptance that the aged do not require, or are not worthy of, the same clinical standards that we apply to everybody else, particularly if they are cognitively impaired.

My colleagues have always resented the accusation that they may discriminate. However, when undertaking Aged Care Assessments in a teaching hospital, they have sometimes expressed their dissatisfaction at my refusal to authorise placement for patients who were obviously delirious, where no attempt had been made to determine the cause. Some have even complained to the administration of the hospital and the administration has tended to agree with them.

Rationing is a reality and probably a necessity where scarce and expensive services are involved. There are strong utilitarian arguments that what is on offer needs to be rationed. These decisions are made at high political levels.

As clinicians, we participate in and facilitate such rationing. Provision of rehabilitation services is a good example. I believe that every person with a disability can benefit from some form of rehabilitation, just as I also believe that there is no clinical situation where prevention cannot play an important role. However, formal rehabilitation is a relatively scarce commodity, and we pick winners: patients who are well on the road to recovery and who have a good functional prognosis. That pretty well automatically excludes anyone with dementia. We should not treat this as an acceptable norm. We should lose some sleep when we refuse it to anyone who could potentially benefit to any degree. We should offer something, not nothing. The principles of prevention and rehabilitation can be applied to some degree in every situation. Nothing justifies nihilism.

While we cannot offer every patient access to scarce resources, we can give them the same access to our clinical expertise that we give to every other patient. Again, nothing justifies our failure to treat every patient with the same diligence that we treat others.

While we cannot influence the rationing decisions directly, we can and must be advocates for our patients both individually and as a patient population.

When our patients have advanced dementia, a significant number of us lose sight of the humanity of the person before us and consider it is not only futile but wasteful to expend scarce resources, such as our valuable time, on these lost causes.

Personhood has long been and continues to be a vigorously debated issue. There are a number of concepts that enter into consideration, ranging from simply being born to having the capacity to think and reason and form relationships. Judgements are made about quality of life from an external perspective by cognitively intact people. I have too often heard, 'the lights are on, but there's nobody home' used as a rationalisation for clinical neglect.

I have seen too many cases where the patient and the life partner have an unbreakable bond and continue to need and to respond to each other when to the rest of us all signs of what we construe as humanity seem to have gone. While the essence of a relationship remains, and that person is important to someone, I think it is wrong to conclude that the spark of humanity has gone.

In one of the country towns that I visit, a man in his 90s insisted on caring for his wife at home. She had very advanced dementia and needed full care that was clearly overwhelming him. He was persuaded to admit her into the local nursing home. I was asked to see her because she was very disturbed and it was almost impossible for the carers to attend to her needs safely. When I saw her, it was impossible to establish any meaningful communication, even with her husband's assistance.

He spent almost all of his time with her at the facility. When personal care was scheduled, he was asked to leave and wait in the sitting room. These attempts at care almost inevitably failed. When I interviewed him, he expressed great regrets about the placement, but recognised that her total care was physically beyond him. There was nothing else he wanted to do, or anybody else that he wanted to be with. I advised the referrer that he should participate in her care, as he had after all been attending to all her needs right up to the day of admission. When he was present, she was calm and cooperative, and with him in attendance, it became possible to care for her, and by extension him, safely and effectively. I think of this as the occasion when I prescribed a husband.

Discrimination is injustice

Ageism

Ageism is systematic discrimination on the grounds of age. It is almost universal. There is very little justification for separating and designating the aged as a group who are different from the rest of the adult population in their need and eligibility for ordinary health services.

The routine and at times prescribed practice of assessing elderly people in the presence of others (as in Geri-Psychiatric Tele Consultations), when it is not usual practice with younger adults, is discrimination.

In Australia, Aged Care is completely disconnected from Healthcare. Singling the aged out for a different range of services, often under different auspices and a different approach to the provision of services, is a form of discrimination. Words like 'age appropriate' and 'homelike' are too often used to justify what is a societal failure of duty of care.

Sexism

The great religions that I am familiar with, Judaism, Islam and Christianity, are patriarchal and paternalistic and are all guilty of discrimination against women. They have always been and continue to be guilty to this day. This is one of the main arguments of feminist philosophy. However, philosophy has also been paternalistic. It is only relatively recently that women have had a voice in the realms of philosophy itself. The voice of half of humanity has only reluctantly been heard. At another time, and in another place even now, I could be put to death for this heretical statement.

Conscience

The United Nations International Covenant on Civil and Political Rights (ICCPR) mentions *conscience* in Article 18.1: 'All human beings are born free and equal in dignity and rights. They are endowed with reason and conscience and should act towards one another in a spirit of brotherhood'.

The strictest judge that we must satisfy is our conscience.

It is interesting to read definitions of the Antisocial Personality Disorder. In a nutshell, such patients lack insight, empathy, and compassion. They have no moral compass, hence no conscience.

Professional ethics

Several of the health professions have codified professional ethics separately.

In its *Ethics Manual* the American College of Physicians[*] outlines the obligations of the physician to society. This includes a responsibility to advocate for the health, human rights and well-being of the public. They point out that physicians have obligations to society that parallel their obligations to individual patients and must conduct themselves as professionals and as individuals who merit the respect of the community.

Specifically, they should help the community and policymakers recognize and address the social and environmental causes of disease, human rights concerns, discrimination, poverty, and violence. They should work toward ensuring access to health care for all persons; act to eliminate discrimination in health care; and help correct deficiencies in the availability, accessibility, and quality of health services, including mental health services, in the community. The manual reminds us that the denial of appropriate care to a class of patients for any reason is unethical.

_____

[*] *ACP Ethics Manual*, 6th edn., 2012.

4

The Healthcare System

Is there a system?

All of the modern Western democratic societies are welfare states. Australia is a welfare state. A welfare state is a concept of government in which the state plays a key role in the protection and promotion of the economic and social well-being of its citizens. Ideally, it is based on the principles of equality of opportunity, equitable distribution of wealth and public responsibility for those unable to avail themselves of the minimal provisions for a good life. This involves a transfer of funds from the state to the key services provided (i.e. healthcare, education, and welfare), as well as directly to individuals ('benefits'). In general, welfare states are either universal – with provisions that cover everybody, or selective – with provisions covering only those deemed most needy.

Esping-Andersen's influential welfare classification* acknowledges the historical role of three dominant twentieth-century Western European and American political movements: Social Democracy, Christian Democracy (conservatism) and Liberalism in defining the character of the welfare state:

1. The Social-Democratic welfare state model is based on the principle of Universalism, granting access to benefits and services to all, based on citizenship. Such a welfare state is said to provide a relatively high degree of citizen autonomy, limiting reliance on family and market. In this context, social policies are perceived as 'politics against the market'. Included in this category are Denmark, Finland, the Netherlands, Norway and Sweden.

2. The Christian-Democratic welfare state model is based on the principle of subsidiarity (decentralization) and the dominance of social insurance schemes.

*   Gøsta Esping-Andersen, 'The Three Political Economies of the Welfare State; The Study of Welfare State Regimes', *International Journal of Sociology*, vol. 20, no. 3, Fall 1990, pp. 92–123.

Countries included in this category are Austria, Belgium, France, Germany, Spain and Italy.

3. The Liberal model is based on market dominance and private provision; ideally, in this model, the state only interferes to ameliorate poverty and provide for basic needs, largely on a means-tested basis. Countries included are: Australia, Canada, Japan, Switzerland and the US.

4. Not clearly classified: Ireland, New Zealand and the United Kingdom.

Although Australia is included under the Liberal model, as a population we have an expectation and belief that what we have here is a Universalist model. We have an expectation that what we have is *entitlements*, rather than safety net provisions. Superannuation is a relatively new phenomenon in Australia. Our expectation had always been that when we retired we would automatically proceed to receive the age pension to which we were entitled, and which would support an acceptable quality of life. Similarly, particularly with the introduction of Medicare we presumed that this was a universal health care system. We have similar expectations for education and welfare.

This is the opening statement on the official Medicare website: 'Australia's health system is world class, supporting universal and affordable access to high quality medical, pharmaceutical and hospital services, while helping people to stay healthy through health promotion and disease prevention activities.'

The most critical issue is funding. Another way of categorising health care systems is by the funding model, which includes:

- Private Insurance Model
- Social Insurance Model, and
- National Health Model

The Health Insurance Commission of Australia tells us, 'Medicare is funded by taxes and the Medicare Levy – a special tax of 1.5% of taxable income (a variation to this calculation may occur in certain circumstances)'. Our model is a combination of all three. There is no discrete health care fund. All the papers and books on the healthcare system that I have studied open with the observation that the funding and management of the Australian healthcare system is extremely complicated.

By whatever classification we look at, the US model rates very poorly against what pertains in other OECD countries and emerges amongst the least accessible and costliest to the government health schemes. From time to time the extreme conservative right attempts to steer Australia in the same direction when our system, for all its faults, is much closer to the best performing countries.

One of the main attractions of the social insurance model is that funds intended for the health system are clearly earmarked. Things have a nasty way of disappearing in General Revenue.

The funds pay for a delivery system that puts policy into operation. Our healthcare system is derivative. It is strongly based on the system that arose in the UK in the 19th century. Over time it has grown and evolved to include new roles for the starting line-up, and new healthcare workers, as well as new activities.

The essential structure has gradually set in concrete. The pre-eminence of the hospital has always been accepted as an unquestionable and unarguable given. This essentially limits the way that reform of the system is or can be addressed. Over time, within the major elements of the system, while new professions and activities were being added, specifically in primary and secondary care, significant activities were being shed.

A modern healthcare system is how all elements of healthcare are delivered to the population. The word system implies that these elements interact as needed in an organised, cohesive, and seamless manner. We assume that it is universal and that all necessary care is delivered to all segments of the population in an efficient and equitable manner based on need.

An ideal healthcare system could be envisaged as a living organism that evolves, grows, and adapts to its environment in a cohesive way. When talking about systems and teams in healthcare, I have used the analogy of the amoeba as descriptive of how the organism reacts to its environment. Whichever pseudo-pod is touched, the whole organism is aware and reacts.

The great Commonwealth/State divide

What we generally envisage as 'the system' is in fact only those elements of healthcare that are controlled by the States. Essentially that is hospital care and the community care that emanates from hospitals. Primary health care and all that is included under that heading is controlled by the Commonwealth and is not an automatic integral part of what we think of as the system.

Aged care, which is also controlled by the Commonwealth is not even considered to be a part of the healthcare system, irrespective of which Department or Ministry it is put under by the Government of the day.

The ageing population: The elephant in the room

The Intergenerational Report 2015[*] released by the Treasury introduced the nation to the concept of the ageing population is if it was a new phenomenon.

The ageing population is the main driver of the shape and content of the healthcare system now and in the future. Its arrival is by no means recent or unexpected. The simplistic conclusion that there will now be a great new burden placed on the diminishing number of working Australians (taxpayers) seemed to offer a rationale for unplanned cost-cutting in the health and welfare systems.

When I specialised in Geriatric Medicine in the early 1970s, one of the first words that I learnt was 'demography', the study of populations. I had gone to England because the specialty of Geriatric Medicine was well established in response to the ageing populations in the UK and Northern and Western Europe. Thereafter, I attended countless local, state, national and international gerontology conferences where the ageing population was always on the agenda. As a WHO consultant, I studied and then brought the demographic trends of their ageing populations to the attention of the governments of several of the nations in our Region.

---

[*] Commonwealth of Australia March 2015, *Intergenerational Report.*

We not only knew that the ageing population was coming to Australia, but we also had living models in the countries listed above of how to cope with age-skewed populations, the like of which was then still a long way in our future.

In Australia, we have been very active in the field of Gerontology and have been major players in the International Association of Gerontology. There have always been good attendances by the Australians from the field at Regional and International Gerontology Conferences. These conferences always offered the opportunity to study the provision of all types of aged care services in the host nations.

My attendances started in the early 1970s. The Scandinavian countries were eye-openers. They had Institutes of Gerontology, Comprehensive Geriatric Services, and outstanding aged care facilities. Our travelling parties were mixed, consisting of gerontologists, geriatricians, Allied health professionals, and representatives of NGOs involved in the Australian version of aged care.

We saw the same things, but we perceived them differently. When we visited a major aged care facility, I would notice that there was a strong health care infrastructure with resources and facilities to provide a significant level of healthcare including continuing rehabilitation. Representatives of the NGOs were impressed by the architecture that managed to cater for the needs of disabled living within attractive homelike environments that facilitated a very agreeable lifestyle. Unfortunately, that is all that they saw. When we returned to Australia, they were much more adept at lobbying and spoke the language that politicians understood.

They did not delve into the funding models. They did not understand the blend of superannuation, insurance and taxation that made all this possible. Hence, to this day, it is only the architecture and the homelike environment that we have emulated.

Successive governments of both persuasions have failed to set up a funding base for the health and welfare entitlements, such as Disability Insurance that we have been taking for granted. What was happening was never a secret. The Bureau of Statistics and the Australian Institute of Health and Welfare have been providing us with high-quality information and expert analyses for many years.

It can be seen that none of the Western nations listed above has gone into an economic meltdown as a result of the growth of the aged proportion of the population, even though most of them had arrived at where we are at present much earlier. They have to varying degrees all been prepared for this growth. We have not.

In terms of health and consequently welfare, the implications have always been clear. The World Health

Organisation has produced a number major scholarly works on the ageing population over the years.

The aged are already disproportionate consumers of health and welfare services. The ageing population brings with it *the era of chronic illness* of all kinds. This calls for a significantly different approach and orientation to the provision of health and welfare services.

In early demographic studies of populations, when looking at the financial implications of the size of different age groups, dependency ratios based on age were developed. The Young Dependency Ratio was: Number 0–14/Number 15–64. The Old Dependency Ratio was: Number 65+/Number 15–64. Several outrageously simplistic stereotypes and generalisations were accepted as valid. These included that all people over 65 were no longer economically productive, were not contributing to society in any useful way, and were economically dependent on the working population and needed (were dependent on) some level of funded support.

What has happened is that the ageing population has been arbitrarily consigned to a population subgroup, 'The Aged', that was no longer automatically eligible to receive the services dedicated to those who still had membership of the Working Age group, but became eligible for services in the segregated 'Aged Care Sector'. This is blatant discrimination concealed by high sounding platitudes.

The people of all ages living in rural and remote areas enjoy a similar form of discrimination in the provision of healthcare. Aged people living in these locations cop the double whammy. Aged people suffering from dementia and mental illness living in these areas hit the jackpot of disadvantage.

The structure of the Healthcare System

The Healthcare System can be envisaged in several ways:

- Levels of Care: Primary, Secondary and Tertiary;
- Types of Care: Primary Care, Curative Care, and Long-Term Care;
- Public health, which is a necessary element of the above Healthcare delivery models.

Unfortunately, because of the Commonwealth/State divide we focus on hospital care (secondary and tertiary care) as the most significant part of the system. I use the word 'significant' advisedly as all elements of the system are important, and I have no intention of undervaluing any of them.

For a sense of proportion, Healthcare must be looked at as a pyramid. The base of that pyramid is unquestionably

Primary Care, which then becomes the obvious and logical Coordination Centre that can ensure appropriate selection of a modality and continuity for the recipients of health services.

The preoccupation with hospitals sinking into lockdown and taking the budget with them would not be of anywhere near the same proportions if the role and potential of the primary care system was recognised and included into a seamless system.

The Commonwealth/State divide makes meaningful reform of the Healthcare System impossible.

I believe that the Commonwealth should be, and behave like, a Funder, not a Provider. That is what pertains in similar countries including Canada and New Zealand.

Primary health care should not only be integral but recognised as the *essential foundation* of the Healthcare Delivery System. Any reform that does not take this into consideration is doomed to fail, as it repeatedly has.

Primary Care, as an element in the structure of the healthcare delivery system, is the only element that serves the whole population, irrespective of age or any other variable. It provides or is involved in the provision of every health-related service.

It is the first point of contact with the system and through triage can determine if the needed service will be provided or referred to another level or be both provided and referred. It provides episodic and continuing care.

It is well placed to monitor and ensure collaboration with all other elements of the healthcare system as well as with other sectors. It is the obvious hub for the clinical information systems.

With the addition of resources, such as access to general hospital beds and infirmary beds in residential facilities, a number of issues currently dealt with only by the tertiary sector could be better managed, easing the pressure on the tertiary sector and introducing economies for the government.

In New Zealand, blessed as it is with a much less complicated system of government, health care is funded by the national government, but delivered by District Health Boards that oversee Primary Health Organisations that deliver primary care to the population. On all the international comparisons that I have been able to access, their system matches or outperforms ours from every perspective.

The Commonwealth in consultation with the States needs to reach consensus on how the system should restructure and operate. As the funder (similarly as pertains in Canada and New Zealand), the Commonwealth would be able to ensure that there were common practices that had to be followed, and national standards that had to be met, and that the States were accountable for the public funds allocated to them.

What we have is a system/structure that evolved in a different era and is perpetuated by a complex arrangement of funding – hence control that hampers, not facilitates, the delivery of healthcare to the population. It largely determines how healthcare is practiced. The structure determines the process. All the States periodically try to reform the system. These attempts are full of good intentions and high-sounding verbiage, but nothing really changes.

Health reform

Whenever reform is proposed, and this happens around every State and Commonwealth election, and whenever government budgets are mentioned, all that ever eventuates is tinkering with the status quo. This basically means keeping the hospitals afloat, and tossing some largesse at a topical current problem, which is almost always a variant of mental health.

In the beginning was the Word, and the Word was Policy (with apologies to the author). *Policy can be defined in a variety of ways. In Blank' s book on the New Zealand Health Policy it is defined as consisting of 'those courses of action proposed or taken by government which affect healthcare institutions, organisations, service, and finance'.*

131

Public policy can be categorised as being of three basic types: regulatory, distributive or redistributive. Regulatory policies limit the discretion of individuals and agencies, or otherwise compel certain types of behaviour. Distributive policies provide services or benefits to particular segments of society. These are generally seen as 'public goods' and they are often based on the notion of entitlement. Redistributive policies represent deliberate efforts by governments to change the distribution of income, wealth, or property among groups in society. This is a central characteristic of the welfare state. Healthcare policies generally encompass all three types, which provides fertile ground for political controversy, particularly in the regulatory and redistributive arenas.

One very major difficulty is that by and large we are confronted by existing policies, which means that reforms and adjustments are made in an unplanned way (what I describe as tinkering). This is scientifically described as incrementalism, which contrasts with rationality. However, policy-making must be a dynamic process to adapt to the changing social, political and technological environment.

There are two major elements that must be continually addressed, namely funding and structure. Efficient and effective function is contingent on both.

There are many barriers to effective reform. I offer the following:

Politicisation and populism

As clinicians, we understand that information of a technical nature, or complex information that requires an educated understanding, must be interpreted. As a population, we are inundated by information that we are incapable of interpreting and lack the insight to recognise this incapacity. We accept persuasive rhetoric and the instruments of propaganda as facts, because we want to believe the person delivering them. What is desperately needed is education, starting from infancy on how to deal with information. In a sense, we lack an adult capacity to evaluate information. Hopefully, this will increase with time.

When a government of any political persuasion organises a review, political bias is inevitable. No government would risk a major review that would advise a radically different course of action to the one that they have chosen. In Australia, we have many highly respected experts in almost every field of endeavour. On the face of it, it would seem simple to assemble a group of such wise and eminent people to examine any issue, if only consensus could be achieved on their selection. Even the mere suspicion of political bias devalues the work of such reviews.

The health, welfare, and education institutions, need to have stability that can withstand political inroads that can threaten their very existence. In the not quiet dim dark past, the Public Service heads of Health and other Departments survived elections and impartially served whichever government was elected. They were respected for their skills and ability, had acquired a large corporate memory, and had and maintained a sense of direction for their department. In more recent times, they have become a threatened species, and I have witnessed a succession of new heads of health departments being appointed based on their service to a political party, rather than their expertise in a given field, in several states where I have worked. This is a great loss of direction and stability. Alas, those of us who recognise this are rapidly (and literally) becoming a dying breed.

Managerialism: It is much easier to teach a clinician management and administration, than a manager a clinical discipline

In the early 1970s I took my family to England to become a geriatrician. An early revelation in England was my first experience with non-medical CEOs. When I departed, The Chief Executive at every hospital in South Australia was the Medical Superintendent.

In one of the Geriatric Hospitals where I worked as a registrar for the longest time, one of the things that we did was to manage many patients who were permanently catheterised. As can be imagined, the complication rate was horrendous. In my previous hospital in Australia we had begun to use silastic catheters as soon as they became available. I discussed this with my Consultant and he had me prepare a requisition with a clear explanation of the benefits. The CEO declined the request. I had a meeting with him to plead the case. He stopped me in mid-flight and told me that the new catheters would cost nine times as much as the old rubber catheters that we were using. No amount of pleading and persuasion could sway him.

This was a stark contrast to my experience at the Repatriation Hospital in Adelaide. We had introduced a hospital-wide system of emergency resuscitation. As medical registrar, I led the team and responded to almost every call, particularly early in the introduction period. The Medical Superintendent, Dr Tom Dearlove, also attended every call that he could. He stood in the background and watched. When all the dust settled, he would take me aside and ask how things went. On one occasion, I told him that the oxygen-giving apparatus was ineffective in the emergency situation. He told me to do some homework and then tell him what I wanted in its place. I consulted with the senior anaesthetist and went to see Tom a few hours later. The new equipment arrived the next day. It was much costlier than the older unit, but Tom had seen for himself and understood the need for something better.

This is but one small example where the head of the hospital displayed clinical insight that overrode any financial consideration. While I have been referring to the 'Medical Superintendent' I must hasten to make it clear that currently I would be more than happy with the term 'Clinical Director', which does not imply gender or any specific clinical specialty.

In later years, with the dominance of managerialism the attitude that I saw in that British Geriatric Hospital so long ago continues to this day. I often rue the day when the medical profession and other health professions lost their rightful place of leadership of our healthcare flagships. As always, I must hasten to point out that I have met and worked with very good non-medical CEOs. The best ones were those who had done the hard yards. They had worked their way up through the healthcare system and had learnt how to use advice and support the health professional leaders in the system.

It takes insight into much more than accountancy and economics to manage health units. I have seen the agony that a Director of Nursing suffered having to make the economies demanded of her by a CEO, who never had any qualms about what those economies meant to the care of the patients in 'his' hospital because his previous experience had all been in the business sector.

One of the things that managerialism introduced was Quality Assurance. This is extremely easy to fudge and tells you very little about the quality of the care that patients and other recipients of our services receive.

I believe that the atoms, the building blocks from which a system is built, are the one-on-one interactions between the patient and the healthcare worker. Beyond that are the basic functional units, or healthcare teams, that operate at the rock face. This is the point at which the quality of the system should ultimately be judged. This is where it is found.

The true business of the healthcare is what these people and these teams do. The higher that we go up into the hierarchy, the further away we get from understanding the purpose of the business and the people who are delivering the service. With managerialism, there is a disconnect between what the face-to-face workers see and aspire to, and how the management perceives the business.

Specialist medical services must be clinically led. In any clinical endeavour, a true leader must be a visible presence throughout his domain. He must be seen to be part of the team at every level and must understand what everyone in the team is doing. He must feel a part of every community in his domain, not just the people in the hospitals or in the health services.

In aged care and in mental health we periodically see examples of institutionalised people in the nominal care of a specialised health service being seriously abused and neglected. This has led to investigations and inquiries where there has been an obvious failure of duty of care by a subordinate clinician who has been punished. If the Director is a senior clinician, that failure can be sheeted home to the Director. A lay Director cannot take responsibility for unacceptable clinical practice.

I would contend that the main goal of a modern hospital is to clear beds for the sake of the budget. This is not a throwaway line. I am a part of a generation that remembers that when someone had major debilitating surgery, they would be in hospital for several weeks, until they convalesced and walked out close to what they had been capable of pre-operatively.

The most damaging effect in this new direction is on the patient population that I care for. They are the victims because they will never be capable of walking out in 4.6 days or whatever is the average for a condition or procedure.

Restructuring the Healthcare System

I believe that the optimal model is based on the development of Area or Regional Services. Most states in Australia have flirted with this concept. Most have decided that central management is the most economically efficient model.

Again, we should make a clear distinction between managing the budget and delivering healthcare. The structure a regional service and the way it functions does not follow the same lines as the flow of money.

The division between Metropolitan and Rural and Remote Services is a formula for perpetuating discrimination and disadvantage. Within subspecialties, particularly Psychiatry creating standalone Psychogeriatric Services is also counter-productive.

What I construe as a region is a discrete area that contains within it the whole range of healthcare services and resources, namely a major tertiary hospital, a psychiatric facility, and specialist clinics and services. Specialist services in hospitals beyond the tertiary, must obviously serve much larger populations.

Within the service, every Clinical Division would be headed up by a senior clinician, supported by dedicated administrative staff and the general administration of the health service. The Clinical Division, say Mental Health, would be responsible for the delivery of their services *equally to the whole population of their area*, be it found in the city centre or the most remote town in the region. Clinicians would be required to travel and provide face-to-face services at all locations. Patients would have equal access to the all centrally located services, including admission. Within the Division sub-specialists would operate in exactly the same way.

Governments of all persuasions and every level talk of Australian values that always include equity and justice, 'a fair go'. As I have postulated, the basic unit of healthcare delivery is the one-on-one clinician/patient relationship and interaction. What governments promise is equal access to that relationship/interaction.

For me, that means that an elderly woman with dementia, whose behaviour makes her unmanageable and a danger to staff and other residents in a rural aged care facility, should have the same (admittedly slim) chance of being admitted into a Psychogeriatric Facility as her twin sister who lives in the capital city. In the same way, a seriously disturbed old man with PTSD that has recently come to light should be able to see a psychiatrist face-to-face, not just at a teleconference with a cast of thousands. We are talking about two types of access here, access to resources and access to people. The common factor is travel. We will never have equal access until travel stops being an obstacle to, rather than a facilitator for access to health care.

In the geographically large, but sparsely populated states, such as South Australia and Western Australia, a major investment in transport makes more sense than buildings and hardware. Having said this, I believe that general practitioners, primary care physicians, should have local access to hospital beds, and long-stay beds.

Clinical Directors would be expected to liaise closely with primary care organisations and networks in their region and would ensure that all clinical encounters were adequately documented and made available to the patient's general practitioner in a timely manner. When a patient is admitted to the regional hospital, communication with the general practitioner should begin from the time of the admission and continue throughout, not just with the discharge summary after the event. The general practitioner is the only one who has a comprehensive knowledge of the patient and can coordinate care and ensure continuity.

Extended Care Services

I believe that the optimal public service framework for the delivery of aged care services is the Regional Aged and Extended Care Service. I see it as a Clinical Division of the overall Area or Regional Service. This Division would be responsible for Rehabilitation and Geriatric Medicine, including Long-Term Care. I discuss this in the next section. This model was in place in Adelaide in the 1990s but did not survive the many reforms that followed.

Residential Aged Care: Where it came from, what it has become, and where it belongs

Aged care has fallen into the Great Commonwealth/State divide and lies seriously wounded

Because I am about to burst into vitriolic prose in my most iconoclastic manner, I will begin with this justification. During my work, I move in the real world. I see people in their homes, in all manner of health care and aged care facilities, and at public meetings and informal gatherings. I meet, get to know, and educate and counsel partners, relatives, and key carers routinely. In this way, I meet many, many able, dedicated, and inspirational people at the workface.

I have argued that the Aged Population has been categorised as a minority group, the 'Aged Dependency Group' (ADG). Like all disliked minorities, it is at risk of discrimination. At greatest risk of discrimination within this group are the Residents of Aged Care Facilities (RACF). Within that habitat, they are isolated from the Healthcare System in its hospital model mode.

When members of the ADG are admitted into a major hospital, they are seen as unwelcome intruders, who interfere with the neat running of the place, and are likely to block a bed (the ultimate sin). They could have avoided this to some extent, by staying in the community. However, should they be admitted to hospital and show any sign of cognitive impairment, they would be at high risk of joining the RACF minority group prematurely, and possibly, if not probably needlessly.

Aged care in Australia

The Australian Institute of Health and Welfare prepared a comprehensive report in 2013–14. The introduction reads as follows:

> The aim of the Australian aged care system is to provide accessible, appropriate and efficient care. It supports the wellbeing and independence of older people through high-quality and person-centred care. Although aged care services are aimed at those aged 65 and over, they are provided on the basis of need, rather than specific age criteria. The system provides a range of services that support older people – and a small number of younger people with disability – in both residential and community-based settings.

> The Australian government provides most of the funding for aged care. As part of the government's on-

going aged care reform, changes have been progressively implemented since 2013. These changes are aimed at ensuring aged care is sustainable, affordable and responds to people's needs. The changes give priority to providing more support and care in the home for all older and frail people (including specifically for those with dementia), as well as better access to residential aged care, and a stronger aged care workforce.

An Aged Care Assessment Team (ACAT) must assess and approve a person before they can access government-funded residential aged care, home care or flexible care services. ACAT provides an approval for both the type and level of care.'

It should be noted that eligibility for the receipt of aged care services is based on *the demonstration of care need*. The needs exhibited by the applicant are the result of disability. Disability does not exist or develop in a vacuum. Disability is the result of impairment. Simply put, it is the result of illness, which is often chronic and continuing. In addition to disability-related needs, they also have needs related to the management of the underlying illnesses, which are commonly multiple. Many of the illnesses experienced by the resident are at an advanced stage and present the most complex problems in management.

The Aged Care Funding Instrument (ACFI) is a resource allocation tool which assesses people in mainstream permanent residential aged care for funding purposes. The instrument is used to determine the level of subsidy service providers will receive for each person in their care. It generates much of the information that is subsequently analysed by AIHW and other interested parties.

All of this data confirms that at the heavy end of residential care we are dealing with the sickest and most disabled people in our population. They should be in receipt of more, not less skilled healthcare than they would if they remained in the community.

Ours must be one of the few long-term care systems for the severely disabled in the world that does not provide significant medical care. Often, residents are made to travel to even see a general practitioner, let alone a specialist. Simple intercurrent illness must be referred to hospital.

The care provided in these facilities touches only a fraction of the care needs.

In 2001, the then Australian Society for Geriatric Medicine issued Position Statement No. 9: 'Medical Care for People in Residential Aged Care Services'. It included this conclusion:

> The Australian Society for Geriatric Medicine believes that the matter of medical service provision in residential aged care requires urgent

collaboration between Commonwealth, State and Territory ministerial portfolios and sections of the bureaucracy that are responsible for primary care; specialist medical services, and residential aged care, in order to establish to whom the reform mandate belongs; and to bring the medical and sectoral stakeholders together to begin the process of reform.

Obviously, nothing happened, and with governments of both persuasions, the Commonwealth, without significant involvement of the health services controlled by the States, continues to provide a very limited service, where a comprehensive service meeting all of the residents' needs is desperately required.

By using the term 'Aged Care' to cover retirement accommodation, serviced accommodation, home care services, low-level residential care, high-level residential care, and secure dementia accommodation, and subsidising businesses and the NGOs to manage every aspect simultaneously, we are doomed to fail.

I would go as far as to accuse the Australian government of failing in its duty of care for these citizens of our nation.

Geriatric Medicine

All the Geriatric Medicine Societies that I am aware of accept that Geriatric Medicine is a subspecialty of Internal Medicine. What then is a distinct specialty?

I maintain that a specialty has a defined patient population that has been societally determined as requiring a special focus of attention.

It has a body of knowledge, based on experience and research, a substantial proportion of which is largely unique to the specialty.

It has special highly developed clinical competencies, techniques, and skills that its practitioners deliver more effectively than non-specialists in the field.

It holds distinct attitudes and values that are required of the practitioner and guide the specialist's approach to clinical practice.

Defined Client Population

- The "old old"
- Constellation of problems
  - Disability
  - Multiple Pathology
  - Cognitive Impairment
  - Social Situation

Our defined client population is largely, but not entirely made up of the 'old old' or more recently 'the oldest old'. What constitutes 'old' is something of a movable feast. In developed countries, people over 65 are deemed old, people over 75 are the 'old old', and the 'oldest old' are those over 85. There is nothing particularly meaningful about these designations, but they seem to give comfort to those of the bureaucratic predisposition and allow statistical games to take place.

Geriatric Medicine

Within a regional service, participating in

- Interdisciplinary Assessment
- Goal-oriented Management
- Rehabilitation
- Resettlement
- Long Term Care

In real life, the patient population is made up of people with a constellation of problems presenting as syndromes rather than individual conditions. I am regularly asked if I am prepared to see a 55-year-old with dementia, or a much younger person with Down syndrome, who appears to be developing dementia. These people have the same array of issues as an 85-year-old with the same diagnosis. I know 90-year-olds who are alert and active members of the community and 50-year-olds prematurely dying of chronic degenerative diseases.

Our unique body of knowledge and our research base is gerontology. Gerontology is the scientific study of ageing. As I have argued above, it has very significant and very necessary contributions from the social and behavioural sciences as well as the biomedical. Geriatric medicine could not be adequately or properly practised in any other way.

As a specialty, geriatric medicine must be integrated into the healthcare and aged care systems. Even a solo private practitioner, such as I, must be involved across both systems in some meaningful way. This is neither difficult nor impossible.

Attitudes and Values

- Respect for the patient's autonomy
- Recognition of psychological, social & cultural influences
- Focus on the family unit
- Provision of services on the basis of asessed need
- Recognition of ageing as a stage of human development

One extremely important way in which we differ from other specialties, probably in common with paediatric medicine, is that we recognise that in the face of complex syndromes with far reaching implications, we must always deal with the family or social unit, not just the patient in isolation as is the practice with almost every other specialty.

With dementia in particular it is impossible to respond adequately to the issues that present to us if this social unit focus is not recognised, understood, and applied.

"Specific" to Geriatric Medicine

- Recognition of differences in patient population:
  - Older
  - Presents with illness differently
  - Cognitive impairment frequently a co-morbidity
  - Multiple problems beyond clinical arena
  - At risk of dysfunction, dependency
- Generally operate in a "bio-psycho-social" framework
- Focus on family, social unit routinely
- Rehabilitation philosophy
- Multidisciplinary approach

The era of super-specialisation

In Australia, Geriatric Medicine entered the arena near the start of the era of super-specialisation. In science and technology, time moves at lightning speed. New knowledge must be accommodated in practice. With super-specialisation in full flight there is a growing need for *super generalists,* who can see the complete picture, the Gestalt in a situation. We have passed the era of the Renaissance man, where an educated individual may know almost all there is to know about nearly everything (like Sherlock Holmes). Our focus must be narrower than this but include knowledge and experience that encompasses the common syndromes seen in old age and the range of therapeutic and rehabilitative responses to the impairments, disability, and handicap that they entail. In essence, all that I have described above.

Our Geriatric Units or Departments should have a strong and visible presence in the major hospitals. They must have the opportunity to admit people in a crisis, to take over patients from other units, as a base for Liaison services, and a venue for teaching and research. Their main activity however should be as the Regional Extended Care Service (as outlined above).

A reminder

British Geriatric Medicine, on which Australasian Geriatric Medicine is modelled was born in residential care.

Dr Marjory Warren (1897–1960) is widely acknowledged as the 'mother of geriatrics', in the UK. As assistant medical officer at the West Middlesex Hospital, in 1935, when the nearby Poor Law Infirmary was integrated into the hospital, she was given the responsibility of caring for 714 chronically ill patients, many of them elderly. Until she took charge of these people, they were invisible to the healthcare service (sound familiar?).

She examined every patient and instituted medical treatment and rehabilitation. Through her work and the many reforms that she introduced, she reduced the number of chronic beds to 240. Many of these patients were returned to the community. The idea that discharge was a reality was a revelation. The lives of all were significantly improved. She published extensively and her writings were of major influence in the birth of the new specialty.

The analogy to the situation in Australia is obvious, as is the task that our specialty must undertake.

An interesting question

If, hypothetically, a State Teaching Hospital ran a High-Level Care annex, would the quality of health care that pertains in equivalent facilities in the Aged Care sector be of an acceptable standard? The answer is Yes and No. A long-term care annex is quite a common arrangement in small country towns. The care there is exemplary from every perspective.

Alas, there have been some notorious examples where the clinical leadership of a Specialty failed completely to provide leadership and establish proper clinical standards, as they did not feel any responsibility for a residential care service operating in their name.[*]

Our place in the system

As specialists and consultants, in private practice or with a right of private practice, we get a choice. We can choose to operate entirely within the Secondary or the Tertiary Sector, or a bit of both.

As 'Super Generalists' dealing with chronic illness we should see our role as supporting and coordinating with Primary Care Physicians. This entails much more than making clever diagnoses and recommendations and withdrawing until the next referral. It entails education and continuing support, in order that the primary care physician can continue caring more effectively for this and similar patients.

This is the role that I have deliberately chosen for myself, and it is described fully in other sections of the book. I believe that when I have made a comprehensive assessment of the patient and offered a recommended care plan that I have entered a Doctor/Patient relationship that is continuing, and at the same time contracted to provide a supporting role to

---

[*] Groves A, Thomson D, McKellar D and Procter N., *The Oakden Report*. 2017, Adelaide, South Australia: SA Health, Department for Health and Ageing.

that patient's general practitioner, also on a continuing basis.

This does not preclude carrying a caseload, but the intent should always be to empower the primary care physician to provide the appropriate continuing care and continuing to make the greatest number possible of initial assessments.

Summation

A fragmented and incomplete system that neglects a very significant proportion of the population obviously desperately needs to be reformed.

In this context, I would define reform as a change for the better. 'Better' can of course be interpreted from many different perspectives. For the government, better is cheaper, and reform is all about cost saving. For politicians, it is about implementing an ideological belief and securing their seat in Parliament. For users of the healthcare system it is about health outcomes.

Genuine reform would require statesmanship and consensus from the government and the opposition. This has been achieved in the past. Is it achievable now or in the future?

Effective systems are built from the bottom up. For a healthcare system, the basic unit, the atom, is the one-on-one clinical encounter. This is what happens at the rock face. This is what the user sees as the system.

The foundation, the control centre, and the principal

workplace is in Primary Care. In coordination with the Secondary Care sector it can reduce the demands placed on Tertiary Care. As the provider of prevention, continuity, coordination, and long-term care it can better health outcomes for the population and ensure greater efficiency in the system.

Primary care is the obvious focus for reform that will percolate through the whole system. This is trickle up rather than trickle down.

The way that the system is managed by the Commonwealth and the States must be cognizant of the fact that it is a dynamic thing that continues to evolve to meet new technologies and other challenges such as the make-up of the population and the emergence of new health issues (remember HIV?).

There should be planned evolution, not periodic revolution to ensure that the system continues to meet the needs of the population.

As practitioners, those operating at the rock face, we all have an obligation to participate in the function, evolution, and reform of the system, and not to assume or accept that we have reached some sort of high point that cannot be improved. The status quo represents the past, not the present, and not the future.

5

The Initial Assessment

Assessment is much more than just diagnosis

The initial assessment of a patient with suspected dementia referred to a geriatrician is of critical importance. It is the entry into the healthcare system which will remain involved for the rest of the patient's life. It is nothing like the response to a referral to a super specialist for a specific problem.

The role that I adopt as a Consultant in Geriatric Medicine, and the way that I deal with the patient presenting with the suspicion of dementia has evolved over many years, and continues to evolve, as I apply experience and new knowledge to the process on an ongoing basis.

I strongly believe that the people presenting to a specialist with presumed dementia for the first time should (*must* if I could enforce it) have a comprehensive assessment irrespective of how, where, and at what stage of the disease they present. For this reason, I treat *every* consultation with a new patient as an exercise in comprehensive assessment and management, irrespective of the specific requests in the referral letter.

This cannot be done in an ordinary consultation, between the management of heart failure and the investigation of a chronic cough.

I consider that the following responsibilities must be met in this clinical encounter:

- Accurate diagnosis of all significant problems, and precise definition of disability & dependency.

- Prognosis: recognition of preventive, remedial, and rehabilitation potential.

- Determination of intellectual capacity & mental illness, including decision-making competence.

- Identification of the family dynamics and social support network, and the impact on the partner/relative/key carer.

- Identification of the patient's and partner's perceptions of needs and possible solutions.

- Formulation of a management plan that can be offered to the patient and the partner, through the referring general practitioner.

- Communication, information, education, and counselling with patient, partner, and the referrer.

- Sharing my knowledge of pertinent services and resources and assistance with access to the most appropriate alternative care options.

- Continuing surveillance and review at the discretion of the referring general practitioner.

The prime objective of the assessment is to identify the cognitive, behavioural, psychological, and functional changes resulting from the neurodegenerative process and their impact on the patient and those around her, most particularly the life partner.

This prime objective cannot be fully met without full consideration of the clinical context.

The referral

As a consultant working in the Australian healthcare system, all the patients that I see have been referred by another medical practitioner, usually a General Practitioner. The nature of the referral often tells me more about the referrer, and the true origins of the referral, than about the patient. Over the years, referrals have come in many forms (all the examples are real):

- Some are irritable and hostile:

  'The family/the nurses insist I get you to see this woman'. The sources of the irritation expressed in this type of referral are multiple. One is indignation that someone other than the patient brings a problem to the practitioner, and has the audacity to suggest that something more than that practitioner's opinion is required.

- Another is resentment that under the prevailing system, the diagnosis must be made by a recognised specialist for the patient to benefit from subsidies under the Pharmaceutical Benefits Scheme, when (this doctor believes) the general practitioner's opinion should suffice.

- These used to be quite common in the good old days when a GP was a godlike Jack of all trades. It proved possible to get under the crust by doing something effective for their patients (see below).

- Some are sceptical:

  'This woman is losing her memory. Her daughter wants you to see her. I did explain to her that there would not be much that you can do, as the cholinesterase inhibitors don't do anything'. This of course assumes that all that the specialist will do is decide to prescribe or not prescribe, as often happens when a specific problem is referred to a super-specialist physician.

- Many are brief:

  'Thank you for seeing Mrs Alice Bloggs aged 84, for an opinion and management. Her family have been noticing deterioration in her memory. Her MMSE was 24/30 when I saw her. This indicates a mild cognitive impairment'. This is an example of a relatively long brief referral.

- The briefest was a barely legible note, fortunately on the practitioner's stationery so that the source could be identified, that said, 'Please see this woman'. I appreciated

the please from this source. It was a sign of
progress.

- A few (and fortunately a rapidly growing
  number) are what is needed, and include
  a full past medical history, a summary of
  observed issues, results of investigations,
  and details of prescribed medication.

What I deduce from this is that many general practitioners find dementia difficult to understand and deal with confidently. In this they are not too different from many specialists, but unlike the specialists, they must deal with the patient and relatives on a day to day basis and can't easily bounce the patient back to anybody else.

The referral reflects the referrer's conceptualisation of the problem. In keeping with most problems that are referred on, the presentation is often simplified to a single symptom or sign. The choice of specialist is made on that basis. If we are confronted with a chronic productive cough, the obvious choice becomes a respiratory physician; angina will be referred to a cardiologist; an abdominal mass must be referred to a surgeon. The history that the referrer feels that the specialist needs to know will not be comprehensive, because it will be deemed irrelevant in the context.

In this conventional way of thinking, dementia generally becomes reduced to a problem with the memory or a troubling behaviour. The choice of specialist is made on this reductionist basis. The patient may be referred to a Memory Clinic if this is an option, or one of several types of specialists in private practice, including neurologists, psychiatrists, geriatricians, and general physicians. The information included in the referral is edited in keeping with the same perception of what the specialist needs to know. This conventional way of conceptualising a problem is often adequate when dealing with a clear-cut disease entity, but is not at all sufficient when we are dealing with a complex chronic illness and a syndrome.

The specialists who accept such incomplete referrals as adequate demonstrate thereby that they too have a limited conceptualisation of what constitutes an adequate referral for what should be a comprehensive assessment.

After completing an assessment, I regularly find myself seeking additional information before I feel that I can produce a meaningful report. The sad thing is that most of the electronic record systems that are now almost universally used in general practice can easily produce a comprehensive referral letter that automatically includes the past medical history, the patient's family history and social situation, and the current medication. Investigation reports are scanned in or delivered electronically. Specialist correspondence is also collected and stored. Everything can easily be passed on.

I must hasten to add, that however peeved I may feel, I never criticise general practitioners or specialist colleagues with patients or relatives. If I have a bone to pick, I will do it face to face (or phone to phone) with that doctor or a clinical supervisor. The patient needs a good relationship with his general practitioner, and I do my best to strengthen and sustain that relationship. I regularly advise the referring practitioner to attribute unpalatable decisions, such as cancellation of a driver's licence or residential placement to me, so that they will not be summarily dismissed by the patient (this is not rare). I have seen an elderly man who progressively went through the general practices in his own town, the regional centre, and then neighbouring towns, because no one was prepared to restore his driver's licence (in this particular instance, a truck licence for which he had no further need).

I have found that most of the initially hostile sceptics amongst general practitioners can be won over if what I find and what I recommend proves to be helpful and beneficial. I do not take offence, but simply recognise the need for education, which is one of the key objectives of my reports.

One of the most important things that we need to understand from the referral is who initiated the process. Even in quite comprehensive referrals, it is mentioned in passing that the family have noticed a change in cognition or behaviour. Referrals from residential facilities mostly cite behavioural difficulties being observed and experienced by care staff and relatives. This is not surprising; the GP is not in a position to see what happens throughout the day in the patient's home or in a facility.

Obviously, there is someone who knows exactly what happens every day at home. It is the partner/relative/or key carer. There are even more people who know what happens in a facility. This yet again raises the question of 'Who is the patient?' As I have argued previously, and will continue to emphasise, the patient is not the single individual who has been referred to us. It is the relationship, the union between the afflicted one and the partner/relative/carer.

Who should assess the patient?

A multidisciplinary team?

Most of the current guidelines on virtually any condition including dementia, recommend that the patient has a multidisciplinary assessment. By implication, this means that a Multidisciplinary Team should see the patient. In this case, as in many others this is accepted as the Gold Standard.

I have organised, participated in, and evaluated many, many teams throughout my career. I have given the topic considerable thought and have written and taught about it extensively. In 1981, the International Year of the Disabled

Persons (IYDP), I had the honour of delivering addresses on this topic around the nation.

Almost every health care worker, who works with or alongside other workers, tends to believe that they are working in a team. There are of course many kinds of teams. It is common for people to compare health care teams to sporting teams. In a soccer football team, there are 11 specialists, skilled at playing a position. None of them, individually, can win a game without the support and assistance from the others. However, it is not the players who determine the strategy that the team employs, it is the coach, and he demands discipline from his team in the implementation of those strategies. Thus, while the team is made up of several 'disciplines', authority to implement practice is not vested in the team, but in a supervisor. There are many clinical teams that match this analogy. Indeed, it is the typical hierarchical model that pervades most health care settings.

Another sporting analogy is that of a tennis doubles team. Each player must support the other, but also must respect his partner's ability and judgement. Each must accept equivalent responsibility when playing the game. Each must make rapid decisions about appropriate responses, without recourse to higher authority, or even consultation with his partner. This is the more applicable analogy for a team in Geriatric or Rehabilitation practice.

I define a multi-disciplinary team as a group of individuals from diverse professional/occupational backgrounds, working cooperatively to achieve mutually agreed goals designed to achieve the optimal outcome for the patient. It should be understood, that the patient and the patient's partner/relatives or key carers *are always an integral part of the team*.

Potential advantages of a Multidisciplinary Team

Range of expertise

When clinical teams are assembled, each member is required to bring some specific skills and capabilities. A typical healthcare team consists of doctors, nurses, and a variety of allied health professionals, including, physiotherapists, occupational therapists, social workers, nutritionists, speech pathologists and many others. Clearly, the combined experience and skill of the team greatly exceeds that of any individual acting in isolation.

Efficiency is achieved through formal processes and role overlap

In most clinical settings, opinions are sought through consultation, usually at the behest of a doctor. The other specialties and disciplines remain uninvolved until they have been consulted via referral. This introduces inevitable delays and leads to breakdowns in communication. In properly functioning teams, core members of the team routinely assess the patient, without the necessity of a referral. This is a standard operating procedure. The results of those assessments are recorded in the communal record, not in discipline-specific notes or items of correspondence.

As workers gain experience in the team, they learn about the roles and capabilities of other members and learn to anticipate when to involve others in the most timely and effective manner.

Improved communication and decision-making.

Good communication does not result from good will alone. It must be facilitated, and must be mandatory, not optional. Communication is both formal and informal. Both should be documented. Formal communication is through the clinical record, working documents, such as Care Plans, and through Case Conferences. Without Case Conferences and collegiate decision-making, a team cannot be said to exist.

The importance of the Case Conference cannot be overstated. This is where the Art is melded with the Science, en masse. This can only happen when there is real respect for the views of every member of the team.

Informal communication is all other communication that is pertinent to a patient that occurs outside the formal settings. Examples include discussions over meals ('shop talk'), and chance meetings with carers and relatives. Where this information is likely to impact on the patient's care, it should be documented in the record, for the attention of the whole team.

Team morale

Good teams are elitist. They strive to be the best in the business, and believe that they are. They are happy in their work, and they enjoy working with the rest of the team. When team morale is high, patient morale is high, and patients do better.

Better after-care, wider networks

Each member of the team brings some unique experience and networks that can be shared and applied to the patient's benefit.

Better relationships with partners and families

I compare a coherent team to an amoeba, a unicellular organism that has no fixed shape and can send out pseudopods to contact its environment. It should not matter which pseudopod, or which member of the team, the patients or carers choose to relate to. All relevant information becomes rapidly known to the whole organism, which can then react appropriately. Different patients relate differently to different members of the team. It is important that they be given the option of choosing the person that they are most comfortable with, provided that that team member understands the implications of what is being communicated, and acts as a conduit to the rest of the team.

Potential problems with Multidisciplinary Teams

Role confusion, insecurity

I mentioned earlier that each member of the team is appointed to a specific role. That role is the prime responsibility and must be fulfilled before there is any extension of the role. Some inexperienced practitioners are not professionally secure in their role and become inflexible and defensive of their 'turf', to the detriment of team function.

Overlap

Role overlap is a valuable development within a team. In addition to specific skills, we bring shared skills, skills that are commonly acquired in the training of other disciplines, and general 'human' skills gained from life experience. We also acquire shared and human skills from our co-workers as we observe their practice and their communications. This becomes a strength within the team. The temporary absence of a team member can be at least partially covered by others assuming some of his or her responsibilities, so that patient care can proceed.

Overstepping

Overlap can become overstepping when someone from one discipline assumes that they have learnt all that there is to know about another discipline, and can completely fulfill all of the roles and responsibilities of another team member.

Imbalance

In some situations, because of availability, one discipline may dominate the team structure. Such teams still assume that they are practicing in a multi-disciplinary mode, but there is no balanced perspective, and usually no incentive to change the situation.

Process confusion

This can arise due to a lack of consensus on goals and inappropriate task allocation. Goals must be arrived at in a collegiate manner, must be clearly defined and documented, and must be attainable through specified activities and be measurable. Vague goals, such as 'making the patient better', are meaningless. Tasks must be allocated to the team member most qualified and experienced to undertake them.

Other structural and process issues

- Confidence and trust in competence

    Team members must respect and trust in each other's capabilities. As in the sporting analogy, you must be ready to pass the ball, confident that your teammate will respond correctly.

- Operational autonomy

    As in the tennis doubles team, each team member must act autonomously and take responsibility for his or her performance, rather than expecting to be supervised at every turn.

- Discrepancies in status, authority

    Multidisciplinary teams are usually made up of people with different levels of formal authority, status and salary outside the team. Within the team, they must be prepared to abandon those differences and accept that everyone is making an equally respected contribution to the attainment of the team's goals, which is ultimately the wellbeing of the patient.

- Sexism

    Many clinical teams are largely made up of women, but headed by men. This reflects longstanding social inequalities and is more prevalent in some societies than others. In an ideal world, people would be recognized for the skill and experience that they bring to bear, rather than any other consideration.

- Lack of processes to achieve decision-making

    In some settings, it is assumed that good intentions and high motivation is all that is required for successful outcomes, and there are no formal processes of communication and decision-making in place.

- Introspection and unjustified elitism

    In some activities, Teams are seen as the Gold Standard – without question the best way to deal with the problem. Some teams become smug and introspective, and fail to study alternative ways of achieving their objectives. They are entirely satisfied with their performance, but fail to produce evidence to corroborate this belief. Teams should always be in a Continuous Quality Improvement mode, ready to analyse performance and outcomes and ready to change if this will lead to an improvement. As individual practitioners, we should all be perpetual students.

- Staff rotation

  In teaching hospitals, there are trainees in every specialty and discipline that must be given opportunity to gain experience in different areas of practice. Even the nominal head of the service is often rotated. At that level, it is assumed and accepted that his skills in this area will be the equivalent of his predecessor. Commonly, the person who established the Service or Clinic was a dedicated pioneer in the arena and brought qualities of inventiveness, enthusiasm, excellent communication, and personnel management skills, that cannot be assumed to be generic within the specialty. I have seen services that have retained the kudos that belonged to that predecessor even though the qualities of that predecessor have not been emulated by his successors. Good documentation can ensure that procedures are carried out to the letter, but cannot guarantee that the spirit of the originator will carry through.

Teams cannot just be appointed. They are organic and must be built. When a key worker makes way for a trainee, it cannot be assumed that that trainee will automatically fit into the team, its operations, and its behaviour.

- The illusion (or is it the delusion) that teams exist where there are none

  Just because a locality may have practitioners of many disciplines operating within it, that does not mean that they constitute a team. There are also teams that fit the following description – 'I have a great team, they all do exactly what I tell them'.

- Waiting lists and slow responses

  Deploying a multidisciplinary team is

expensive and cumbersome. This is fully justifiable and unquestionably the gold standard in such areas as neurological rehabilitation, but is it justifiable in the initial assessment of a very common problem? It is doubly frustrating when all that results from the assessment is simply a pathogenic diagnosis.

- Isolationism

  Little effort is made to include the general practitioner, the one who knows most about the patient and who will have to implement any plans developed by the team. There are many practical reasons for this. Many years ago, when I set up a rehabilitation unit, I issued invitations to the patient's general practitioners to attend our weekly case conferences when their patient was being reviewed. Very few took up these invitations. It was explained to me that they simply could not afford to spend the time away from the practice. I, and everyone else at the case conference was salaried. It reflects a, if not the most important failing of our Healthcare 'System': the failure to

comprehend that primary care is the base
and control centre of any true system.

A Geriatrician?

The Stroke Rehabilitation Team model is without doubt the
Gold Standard, but the Memory Clinic Model is not.

Referrals to a Stroke Rehabilitation Team are all
elective, and there is an orderly process of admission, where
priority for admission is well understood.

Referrals for dementia assessment are not all 'elective'.
Families find themselves suddenly confronted with a
disturbed member, and disturbing behaviour and anxiety
about the day-to-day safety of a spouse, partner, or parent.
I need not point out that this is something that happens to
many people every day somewhere in the area that we serve.
The incidence of disabling stroke, while not rare cannot be
compared to this.

I believe that it is not only unjustifiable on any
economical evaluation, but that it creates bottlenecks
that make Teams unable to respond to the commonest
presentations of dementia that are in effect crises.

In the community, of necessity diagnoses of dementia
must be made by specialists working alone or with very
truncated teams where the relationship is informal. As

I have explained previously, I believe that this is a role for a Super-Generalist, a one-man multidisciplinary team equipped with more than basic knowledge of the areas of expertise contained within real teams and how this expertise can be engaged and applied in the best interests of the patient and life partner. Essentially this generalist must have the capacity to fulfil the obligations listed previously.

In stroke rehabilitation, the prime focus is predominantly on physical disability. There are many allied health specialties that can make a major individual contribution in highly technical ways. The outcome is usually positive with an increase in function and independence, and there is a clear-cut end to the intensive phase of the process.

When we are dealing with a syndrome such as dementia, where emotional and psychological problems are to the fore, the one-on-one doctor/patient relationship becomes of critical importance. In parallel, a similar relationship must develop between the doctor and the partner/relative/carer. In the classical multidisciplinary team model, in the Memory Clinic the most meaningful one-on-one relationship that develops may be with a nurse or social worker, who can convey impressions to other members of the team including the consultant. The consultant is then dependent on witness evidence, without his own impressions and gut feelings, and never develops a deep relationship with either the patient or the partner.

In dementia, there is no easily definable end. The disabling disorder is progressive and will need to be addressed until the death of the patient.

As discussed above, Teams must be built. I was always in the happy position of being able to choose the members of my teams. In the early days, this involved considerable negotiation and exertion of influence to prevent routine circulation of members of different disciplines through my units. I chose people who apart from qualifications had the personality attributes to work within a tight team, and whose findings and opinions could be trusted without question. I understand that hospitals must teach and train and give people experience in the many different work situations that a hospital presents. However, a Memory Clinic, just as an elite Stroke Rehabilitation Unit, is not a starting place for beginners. Too much depends on how they perform.

As an individual super-generalist, I would be happy to pit myself against any Memory Clinic. I have worked in several. I will be saying some harshly critical things about screening tests later in this chapter. Even something as dangerous and useless as the MMSE can have some value when you perform it yourself, and don't simply accept a score from a practice nurse, a medical student, general practitioner et cetera.

Even though my consultations are very long, they represent enormously better value for the taxpayer than the services of a Memory Clinic. Add up the costs of the multiple clinical contacts, the meeting time, and the cost of the inevitable tests and investigations that follow.

I am prepared to compromise and admit that my most effective and satisfying consultations in the rural areas have been as part of a two-practitioner Assessment Team. In forming such a team, my current first choice would be a Social Worker. I have also had similar job satisfaction working with senior nurses with aged care experience, and after only limited contact, with Nurse Practitioners, I could see them as able to play this role.

Where should the patient be seen?

It will come as no surprise that I believe that *in this context* patients should be seen where they lie, particularly when there are disturbing behavioural issues, and where a change of accommodation is in question.

The issues that confront us always occur in a context, which includes the patient's situation in locational terms. The patient's environment is a significant factor in the creation and perpetuation of the problems that lead to a referral for consultation. We are often being asked to make decisions that have extraordinarily far-reaching implications for the rest of the patient's life. The consultant's comfort and convenience becomes a very secondary consideration. Where future accommodation comes into question, there is no justifiable alternative to a home visit, or at the very least an examination of the home and consultation with people who have participated in the care of the patient in that setting, by someone with the capability and experience to understand what they are observing and learning.

My modus operandi

My modus operandi has evolved over many years. It has not stopped evolving, but in recent years the changes have been refinements to accommodate new knowledge.

I approach every new patient in every situation, home, clinic, hospital, or residential facility, and whatever the reason for the referral, in an *identical systematic manner.*

When I was a registrar, I was answerable to my clinical mentor, Dr Peter Last, a consummate physician. He introduced the Problem Orientated Medical Record to our hospital, and insisted that it be strictly adhered to with every admission. Facing him in the morning after a hard night, could be quite daunting if our admission records were deficient in any way. As his registrar, I policed and enforced his standards. They have been my standards throughout my professional life.

Treating everyone with the same care and consideration as anyone else is a simple way to demonstrate a true adherence to the ethical principle of justice.

The patient interview

Irrespective of the reason for the referral, I routinely do a comprehensive assessment and work to a protocol that I have evolved (and continue to evolve) over the years. This could be described as 'opportunistic' screening.

Engaging, establishing rapport

In clinics or rooms, I always meet the patient in the waiting room. In hospitals or aged care facilities I meet them at the bedside and escort them into the consulting room or wherever else I may be conducting the interview. I try not to see patients in wards or bedrooms. There is always somewhere that it is possible to meet the patient on more normal terms, even if they must be taken there in a wheelchair. I do not like to have a desk between me and the patient. We need a writing surface but the corner of a desk or table will suffice.

We should be aware that not only is the patient anxious about the interview, they see us as aloof authority figures, who do not consider them as our equals in any way. They are sceptical that with our background, which they assume to be privileged, we cannot understand what it means to grow up on a farm (a working class suburb) and live most of your life in Woop Woop (rental accommodation in a working-class suburb).

Wherever I meet the patient, I introduce myself, shake hands and greet the patient respectfully by surname, and any partners/relatives/carers who have accompanied the patient. This often surprises some of the more disturbed patients, but it is rare for them not to respond to this friendly courtesy. This is the first step in establishing rapport and setting the scene for the interview.

Humour comes easily to me, and the more resistive, hostile or anxious the patient is, the more I rely on it. This involves banter and mild self-deprecation (e.g. 'Sorry I'm late, I'm hopeless at keeping appointments unless I write them down', 'I forget people's names as soon as I meet them'). I could probably be a successful stand-up comedian if I needed another occupation. On a home visit, I look for clues to the person's achievements and interests ('Wow, I get to meet a real star of country and western music'. 'Are all those paintings your work?' 'I see you're a Port supporter. That was some game last week!' [all real examples]). This way they see me as a real person, capable of understanding them and their lives. I don't get described as 'a cold fish', like some of my eminent colleagues.

I pride myself on my ability to establish and maintain rapport with almost every patient that I am asked to see. It is now rare for me to fail, nearly always in the context of restless delirium, but it was not always thus. I have learnt how to do it, and what can be learnt can be taught.

Separate interviews

I believe that separate interviews should be the standard, mandatory procedural norm in the assessment of cognitive impairment. There are many parallels with legal process. We must be cognisant of the legal and ethical reality that all people have the right to be heard privately and confidentially without risk of influence or duress.

In an assessment, we are gathering information that will inform decisions and determine courses of action with serious and far-reaching consequences. This information may literally become evidence that will inform legal decisions. If the process of gathering the information is flawed, then the evidence, decisions, and actions that flow from it may be equally flawed.

The law starts with the presumption that people have mental capacity until proved otherwise. In the context of proven or seriously suspected of cognitive impairment, and delirium, this is not the starting assumption that we should apply in this context. We know or can safely assume that the patient's perception and comprehension of the situation is seriously inaccurate. Furthermore, there is no, or very limited capacity to evaluate information rationally.

We need to understand what the information that we obtain from different sources is comprised of. From the patient, we get *perceptions and beliefs*, that may need to be validated.

When I interview relatives and carers, also privately, what I want from them is *observations*, which are more likely to be objective than the patient's perceptions and beliefs. At the start of an interview many partners and relatives provide assumptions and rationalisations not observations. For example, when I ask the question, 'Does your mother seem to be depressed?' The answer is often, 'Of course she is depressed. She used to be a teacher, now she can hardly read'. That answer is an *assumption and rationalisation*, based on how the daughter would feel if she found herself in the same predicament. I explain this, and then ask, 'Does she mope about, does she cry, does she complain that her life is not worth living?' It is only when we get to actual observations that we can make an accurate judgement.

I see numerous examples where important conclusions have been based on very poor evidence gathered by a process that is politically correct but clinically flawed.

The fact that I will interview the patient alone first is

explained to the referrer when the appointment to see me is made.

Most relatives who ask to be present are doing so out of genuine concern, and can be easily persuaded of the wisdom of the separation, and sometimes agree to find some excuse to leave the room once rapport and communication has been established (e.g. 'Sorry mum, I must dash off to the toilet, you just keep talking to the doctor').

Where relatives insist that they must be present, I remind them that I will interview them after I have interviewed the patient and will take their views into consideration. I point out that I don't necessarily believe everything that I am being told. This is a common anxiety and easily allayed.

When relatives still insist that they must present, and will not allow the interview to proceed otherwise, and where there are obvious issues with family dynamics, the possibility of conflict about inheritance, or suspicion of some form of elder abuse, I refuse to see the patient on their terms, and advise them to seek a consultant opinion elsewhere. Where a legal authority has requested such assessments, I report the reasons for not being able to undertake the assessment back to that authority.

In a clinical assessment, the interview begins with engagement as the starting point of a clinical practitioner/ patient relationship. One very important reason for seeing the patient alone initially is to determine if they can be engaged.

It is important to 'get into the patient's head', to try to visualise the situation from the patient's perspective. Almost every patient presenting for a cognitive assessment is anxious, fearful, suspicious, and hostile to varying degrees. These feelings are multiplied in a disturbed patient, and the fear and hostility may result in overt aggression in self-defence.

Successful engagement requires us to present an aura of calm, friendliness, and sympathy. This is possible in most situations, but when patients are delusional and extremely anxious, it may be necessary to resort to medication to facilitate engagement. The patient must be persuaded that we are people that he can trust and who will respect his confidentiality. This is not possible in front of an audience (e.g. in a teleconference with a psychiatrist, mental health nurse, and social worker at one end, and the patient, a relative and a mental health worker at the other end). Other people, who will participate in the patient's care can, and must be introduced at a later stage.

Rarely in my experience, some very anxious patients will not even commence the interview without their supporting relative or carer. Even then, once rapport is established, it is often possible to engineer a discreet withdrawal. More commonly, people want the partner/relative because they cannot remember   their medical history, and are anxious not give the wrong information. They are easily reassured (sometimes repeatedly throughout the interview).

I now find it very difficult to question the patient, or a relative, as freely as I do when seeing them separately, and this affects the quality of the consultation. I only rarely agree to work with these constraints, usually in situations where an urgent decision is needed, and the consultation cannot be deferred or directed to someone else.

There are ethical and legal objections to joint interviews on grounds of privacy, confidentiality, and duress, as I have discussed previously.

It is interesting that many of my learned colleagues believe that in doing so I am essentially wasting time. They tell me with a certain degree of patronisation that they can make a confident diagnosis of dementia and its type in a 30-minute consultation, and that they do not need any additional evidence from relatives. I have had quite intense arguments with psychiatrists when I have questioned the evidence for their conclusions when they have interviewed elderly people as couples, when they routinely interviewed other, younger patients separately and confidentially apart from rare ventures into couple therapy.

After seeing patients in hospital or residents in an aged care facility I then interview carers who are very familiar with the patient in that setting. I like to speak to those who have frequent daily contact with the resident.

The management of dementia in residential facilities takes a battering in the media. While I agree that it could and should be done much better, the one-on-one care delivered by the lowliest carers on the totem pole is often inspirational.

I am not an enthusiast of tele-conferencing for reasons other than first aid, stop-gap, or psychotherapy and follow-up, because under the rules there are obligatory witnesses at both ends that precludes a confidential one-on-one interview. On one occasion, I saw an elderly woman in a country town who had a long history of anxiety and depression. I was the first person she had ever told of having been sexually abused by a close relative when she was a small child. Her attempts to report this to her mother resulted in blame and chastisement, and she did not confide in anyone thereafter. The issues had been very real to her throughout her life and had begun to trouble her more and more severely in recent times. She cried throughout the interview. I made a confident diagnosis of PTSD. I arranged for her to be reviewed by a psychiatrist to try to get her access to counselling and psychotherapy. The psychiatrist interviewed her by teleconference. A mental health nurse accompanied him. The patient was accompanied by her daughter and a local mental health worker.

The patient did not complain of anxiety or depression at the interview. She in fact said very little about anything, and the psychiatrist concluded that she was being adequately managed with an antidepressant, and that the anxiety that I had referred to was caused by me, because I had interviewed her without her daughter being present in support.

In some settings, I am regularly told that the patient won't be able to tell me anything. Sometimes that is literally true; when they are completely obtunded and when they have minimal verbal communication. Much more often, a great deal can be learnt from the patient. Students and trainees are regularly amazed by how much information I glean from 'hopeless' patients. It must not be forgotten that much valuable communication is non-verbal. A great deal can be learnt from simple observation.

Separation of interviews allows me to focus entirely on the patient's recollection, perceptions of symptoms and issues, perceptions of functional capabilities, and attitudes towards interventions that may become necessary. The comparison of the patient's views and perceptions with those of a partner/relative or key carer can make the difference between diagnosing, or not diagnosing the existence of dementia.

At the completion of the patient interview, I ask the patient for permission to interview their relative(s). This is very rarely refused. Even patients who are hostile towards their relatives, or suspicious of a conspiracy generally consent. There have been some instances where the patient has been severely depressed and full of guilt and shame, where I do not persist with my request. When patients refuse permission, I honour this refusal. The refusal of itself is a telling piece of clinical information.

One very real and practical consideration is that patients can become extremely anxious when the informant interview takes more than a few minutes. Many of my patients cannot simply be sent off to the waiting room to read a magazine. In my private practice, my wife, who assists me, comes and chats with the patient while the relatives are being interviewed. She is adept at keeping people calm and entertained. If the relatives have come with children, as a very experienced teacher, she keeps them entertained as well. She often adds important observations to my fund of information.

An arrangement like this could be a very valuable addition to a formal Memory Clinic.

On my rural visits, I regularly work with a local supporter who, in the past was a member of the Aged Care Assessment Team, or someone involved in Aged Care or Dementia Care. Alas, 'reform' of the aged care assessment system has deprived the teams of the ability to contribute very significantly to the well-being of aged people in their locality. I interview the patient, while my co-worker talks to the family. A great deal of useful information is exchanged in these talks. The workers learn of the family concerns and because of their local knowledge can explain what resources are available in the community and how they are accessed. When I have completed my interview with the patient, we change places, and I conduct an informant interview, while the co-worker talks to the patient. During the day, we exchange information and have informal case conferences.

I have discussed this point with many colleagues, and I am aware that routinely seeing people separately is not a common practice. Some say that it is not necessary because they can learn everything that they need to know by interviewing the patient and partner together. Some say that there is simply not enough time in their schedule to do this routinely, and only do it when they think there is a particular indication.

I have met and addressed many Carer Groups. I am often asked how patients are assessed and diagnosed. I describe my routine practice. Many relatives have said that they wished that the people who had dealt with them had operated in a similar manner. One very distressed wife told me that she was shown the report that another geriatrician had sent to the general practitioner. In the report, the geriatrician commented that the wife contributed very little to the interview. She was devastated. She had had numerous concerns but was not prepared to state them in front of her husband, because she believed that he would have been very hurt, and she did not want to do that, no matter what her own difficulties were.

The assumption that because one is a very experienced practitioner, one can always tell when a specific issue must be raised, or an assessment instrument used is dangerous. There are people with highly developed social skills and daunting personalities ('Social Facade') that make people hesitant to question their cognitive state, or even their sanity. I suspect that few people can match my experience, yet, there have regularly been people that I only diagnosed because I adhered to my routine practices, including doing cognitive screens routinely, and interviewing relatives and carers routinely.

I am reminded of a protest from a number of experienced Case Managers, when I insisted on cognitive screens as an obligatory part of entry assessment into a very large Home Support Program of which I was the Clinical Director. They too knew when assessment was necessary and when it wasn't. The objection was withdrawn on review of the entry process.

The case-taking protocol

I cannot stress strongly enough that the initial assessment must be structured and adhered to irrespective of any other consideration. The conventional approach is guided by several dangerous starting assumptions. We may assume that that when the patient can achieve a high MMSE score there is no significant cognitive impairment and that a comprehensive assessment can be put off for months until a lower score creates eligibility. Furthermore, that other manifestations begin to appear in an orderly sequence when the MMSE score indicates greater severity, even though the literature tells us that depression, a psychotic episode, or delirium may precede the diagnosis of dementia by months and years.

I allocate 90 minutes for an initial assessment.

I always try to start with a clean sheet. Patients come with reputations. The referral is often triggered by behavioural or situational crisis, where stress levels are very high and there is emotional conflict.

In advanced dementia, which is commonly when patients present for the first time, there are often major issues affecting family dynamics and relationships with carers. In hospitals, where staff are often inexperienced in dealing with disturbed patients (with or without delirium) they will see them as disruptive, demanding and attention seeking. In residential facilities, the patient's behaviour and utterances may seem to have malicious intent. It is easy to accept the prevailing judgement as the reality, and respond in accordance with this, usually mistaken belief.

I believe that the protocol is essential in the assessment

process. It covers all aspects of the patient's symptomatology, behaviour, function, and social situation. It ensures that my assessment is truly comprehensive and keeps me anchored and disciplined in adhering to it. At the end of a heavy day, there is often the temptation to take shortcuts, but I understand what this would cost in the integrity of my assessment. It takes as long as it takes.

Assessment Protocol

- Recollection of Past Medical History
- Current Concerns
- Systematic Somatic Inquiry
- Psychiatric and Social Inquiry
- Accommodation, Basic and Instrumental Activities of Daily Living
- Cognitive Testing
- Information Interviews, Other Information

It gives structure, consistency, and reproducibility, and some numerical baselines to the consultation. It has a series of landmarks and does not have to be applied slavishly in order. Often a patient who has been difficult to engage begins to talk. What he is saying may be out of sequence but is very relevant and it can be easily located in the protocol. It is then a very simple matter to return to the earlier sections that have not yet been completed.

Use of the protocol saves considerable time. A simple 'X' may be all that is required, but it is proof to me that I have asked the question. Any item can be expanded upon as appropriate and necessary.

Students and trainees often observe that I can elicit a great deal of information from very unpromising sources, such as a disabled old man with dementia in an aged care facility, who so rarely talked to anyone that people assumed that he had no opinions. There is no secret formula to disclose. What I bring to bear is structure, my time, and communications skills.

Documenting the protocol

The protocol is a four-page document divided into four sections: Physical Health; Psychiatric and Social Inquiry; Living Arrangements, ADLs and IADLs; and Informant Interview. There is space in each item for notes. If this space is insufficient I add another page.

It seems that I differ from the medical stereotype, in that patients are fascinated because I use a fountain pen and I have very neat writing. I can make notes very quickly usually without slowing the flow of our interaction. In the distant past when I was a medical student, we all learnt to take copious notes with a speed that matched a court reporter. I include a lot of verbatim quotations in the patient's own language, e.g. 'my son wants to dump me in a nursing home'. These quotes reflect the patient's concerns, fears, and temperament. I believe that their inclusion in some of my reports gives the recipients of these reports a better understanding of the situation. Certainly, I have had a lot of feedback to that effect.

The occasional suspicious patient has asked me why I am writing everything down. They usually accept the explanation that I see a lot of people, and I must be very sure that I will remember everything of importance and not confuse one patient with another.

Communicating with the patient

The language of medicine

When my wife and I don't want people to know what we are talking about, we switch to Ukrainian. Suddenly, no one can understand. What many people in the healthcare professions have forgotten, or simply do not realise, is that during their training they learnt a foreign language, a language that is foreign to lay people. Even well-read and educated people don't understand this language, yet we assume that the elderly person who has been referred to us because someone suspects that they have a cognitive impairment, will somehow magically understand what we are talking about.

When he asked what was happening to his wife, a spouse had the amyloid hypothesis earnestly explained to him by a specialist colleague.

Perhaps the most spectacular example of this was when I did a stint of psychiatry as a resident. The Chief Psychiatrist, who could most kindly be described as a strange man, liked to have junior medical staff sit in while he interviewed patients. On one occasion, peering over his half glasses he asked a confused elderly man, 'Do you ever experience auditory or visual hallucinations?' The response most closely resembled, 'Huh'? This was recorded in the case notes in his spidery hand as, 'No auditory or visual hallucinations'.

On one occasion, when I was a Medical Registrar, I brought a surgeon to see one of my elderly patients who had a suspected bowel obstruction. The surgeon asked, 'When did you last have your bowels open'? The old chap, looking very worried, stammered, 'I've never had any operations'. I stepped in and asked, 'When did you last have a shit'? 'Oh' he said, 'a couple of days ago'.

Where we are dealing with people with cognitive impairment, or simply people who have adapted to a chronic condition, however dysfunctionally, we must ask direct questions. 'If you don't ask, you will never know'. We are not in a court of law where leading questions must be avoided at all costs. Certainly, the patient should be given the opportunity to express himself in his own words, but often leading prompts are needed to arrive at meaningful answers.

Maintaining rapport

From the outset, we must address the patient with respect and dignity irrespective of the circumstances. When dealing with a disturbed or cognitively impaired patient, maintaining rapport is a continuous process. It can change abruptly and unexpectedly. This calls for close monitoring of the patient's levels of stress, his ability to maintain attention and concentration, and his ability to comprehend what is going on, and what we are saying and asking. It is important to avoid making our interview a quasi-legal interrogation. This would stress anybody. We must also remain calm and unflustered, irrespective of the provocation that we may confront. We must know when to back off and start again. We must not show that we are pressed for time. We must not seem judgemental or biased.

As I have noted above, I rely heavily on humour that shows me to be an ordinary friendly and fallible human being. This diffuses tense situations and minimises the threat that I may seem to present as an authority figure. This is learnt and quite calculated behaviour on my part. Again, as I have stated above I deem it a major failure if I cannot establish and maintain rapport with even the most disturbed patients.

Commencement

As stated above, I always meet and greet the patient in the waiting room. I refer to her by surname and introduce myself to her and those with her. We shake hands. I explain that I will interview the patient alone first and will then speak to the family. The family at least already knows this. It is made clear that this will be the format when the appointment is made. The approach in hospitals and aged care facilities it is very similar.

In the consulting room, or at the bedside, I explain that I am a geriatrician, a physician (not a psychiatrist) who specialises in the care of older people. I explain that I will undertake a rapid but comprehensive general assessment of all aspects of her health (which is the literal truth, irrespective of what is requested in the referral) to ensure that we (the GP and I) are doing everything that we should be doing to keep her as well as we can, for as long as we can, so that she can continue to enjoy her life in her chosen environment for as long as possible.

I explain that, to enable this I will do a general assessment of all aspects of the patient's health. I also explain that I will be using a structured protocol (not literally in those words) and that some of the questions and simple tests (cognitive screens) and many of the things that we will talk about, will not necessarily be immediately relevant to them.

With necessary adaptations, I do something very similar in every setting.

The patients who present are almost invariably anxious, and often feel frightened and threatened by what is happening. With some, the question, 'What's all this about'? recurs throughout the interview and requires the same reassurance each time (good evidence of short-term memory loss). They are afraid/suspect that I am there to prove that they are going mad, and that this is all part of the conspiracy to place them in a nursing home or take away their driving licence. My introduction is designed to defuse this anxiety.

Past medical history from the patient's perspective

I ask this even if there is a complete Past Medical History in the referral letter. This is not always the case, and some GPs (fortunately he a decreasing number) do not consider this relevant information. This is one of the practical ways that one can test episodic memory, and should alert us to the likelihood that much of what the patient says will not be strong factual evidence.

It is common for patients with a horrendous PMH to tell me that they have been very lucky with their health and have never had a serious illness. One such woman, who told me that she had only ever been in hospital to have babies, told me that she had been very lucky and was remarkably healthy for her age. She had had a coronary bypass and a below knee amputation.

Current concerns. Whose problem is it?

I ask the patient if they have any current concerns about their health, or any other issue that is troubling them. By then, many have already told me that they have been 'very healthy', 'very lucky', or 'great for my age' regarding their health and simply reaffirm this, and then the preface their answers to questions in the next section with this response repetitively.

Then I ask the patient if she understands why her doctor referred her to see me. Some are baffled, given that they have no problems and are so well, and are surprised to learn that they have been referred to a specialist. I reassure them that we will solve this mystery together.

Some, who have remembered that they were seeing a specialist, have been surprised to find that I was not the podiatrist, the dentist, or the hearing aids specialist; and on one occasion when I was wearing dark clothes, the priest.

A very significant proportion of the patients say that they do not know why they have been referred but have acquiesced to family concerns and pressure. Some say that their relatives feel that there is a problem with their memory, but they do not really agree that this is the case.

Some are openly hostile and anxious because they fear that seeing me is the prelude to placement, and that there is some sort of conspiracy in which their family and their doctor are complicit. I reassure them that this is very unlikely given what I know about the doctor, and anyway I always try to begin with a blank slate and form my own opinions. Some patients who did not seem anxious at the outset, have confided in me at the end of the interview that they had been very worried about what was to take place and were pleasantly surprised that I had been friendly and helpful and that their worst fears had not come to fruition.

Very few of the patients that I see are the instigators of the referral. Many of those who are, turn out to be 'the worried well', who are very anxious or depressed. As noted above, in the community, the referral is almost invariably generated at the request of a relative. In residential facilities, it is mostly care staff, and sometimes relatives that request a geriatrician's opinion.

The medical convention is that it is the patient who has the problem, and consultations are undertaken based on this assumption. However, as discussed above, the patient is not the one that has identified a problem and requested that it be addressed, and often has denied the existence of any problem. This point seems to be lost on much of the medical profession. I have already contended that our patient is not only the individual before us, but the patient/partner union. Similarly, it is often (usually?) not the patient who has the problem that we are expected to address. It is the non-afflicted partner.

Systematic somatic inquiry

I deliberately commence with issues that are clearly the sort of health problems that patients bring to and talk about with doctors. This is non-threatening and allows rapport to develop. I perform physical examinations as necessary in each section.

The structure and content of the somatic inquiry

This inquiry is structured in terms of the major systems. Within each section I specify the questions that must be asked in every instance. One of the aims of this inquiry is to discover which of 'The Giants of Geriatrics'* apply. It should be remembered that these Giants not only co-exist, but also play a significant part in the aetiology of the others. In brief, the Giants are:

- Immobility
- Instability

---

* Isaacs, Bernard (1992) *The Challenge of Geriatric Medicine*, Oxford University Press.

- Incontinence

- Intellectual Impairment

As I have repeatedly stated before, dementia occurs in a context. Co-morbidities are a very important part of that context. Therefore, another very important goal is to determine what role they are playing in the patient's presentation.

A prime example is Diabetes. This is very commonly found in this patient population, even if the patient does not remember that he has it. Diabetes per se is a risk factor for cognitive impairment, particularly through the long-term complications. These complications can cause or contribute to several, if not most of the other Giants.

This segment is organised as a checklist. It gives a reasonably comprehensive overview of somatic issues, with emphasis on the common geriatric problems, but covering all co-morbidities. Any item can be explored further. I will touch upon some of the commonly encountered issues.

Cardiovascular system

- Angina

- Effort dyspnoea

- Peripheral oedema

- Palpitations
- Claudication

As in all the succeeding sections, the words above are aids memoire for me, and are not the actual words that I use with the patient. The answer often needs to be expanded and explored. For instance, the way that the patient describes chest pain may be more typical of an oesophageal than cardiac cause, and this will be pursued in detail in a subsequent section.

I ask the patient if they ever experience the feeling that their heart is beating very rapidly or irregularly. I routinely feel the pulse after asking this question. I estimate that I discover a new case of atrial fibrillation in about every 10th patient that I see. Another way of looking at this is one every day that I spend at a rural location. It should not be forgotten that this is not a random selection of the general population, but people who have had a lot of contact with the healthcare system. The significance of this finding in the context of dementia is obvious.

Intermittent claudication is another previously undiagnosed problem that I find periodically.

Some conditions are very difficult for patients to describe because they do not have the language for it. Claudication is an example. Waiting for someone to volunteer this diagnosis is futile. The symptoms must be clearly described for it to even emerge as an issue. Obviously, this is a question that must be raised at least with every diabetic and I regularly find previously undiagnosed patients with peripheral vascular disease.

Respiratory system

- Smoking
- Cough
- Chronic Respiratory Disease

There are not too many surprises under this category, but the lasting damage that smoking does is repeatedly demonstrated. Several widows, particularly War Widows, who have never smoked, have told me that they were surrounded by heavy smokers for most of their life.

Gastrointestinal system

- Appetite
- Weight
- Eating/Dental
- Reflux
- Dysphagia

- Nausea/Vomiting
- Abdominal pain
- Bowel pattern

This is a high yield area.

Loss of appetite and weight loss are very common and are frequent vegetative signs of depression. Quite massive weight loss, inexplicable by any other cause, is regularly found in association with depression.

Dental and oral problems are common. It is not unusual to see people who explain that they take their dentures out so that they can eat. The diet can be very poor because of oral pain and difficulty chewing.

Dysphagia is an important symptom and is often unnoticed and undiagnosed. In advanced dementia, it is a very ominous sign because of the risks associated with inhalation.

Oesophageal reflux can present in a variety of different ways and for different reasons and needs to be evaluated.

Constipation could easily be added to the list of Geriatric Giants because it is so common. What is much less common, but of major importance is faecal incontinence. One way that this comes to light is when the patient response to the question, 'Are your bowels regular?' with the answer, 'Too regular'. On further questioning they complain of frequent bowel motions and faecal urgency, which may then be followed by incontinence. They are reluctant to talk about it and may have been covering up their 'accidents' to keep it secret from their carers.

Urogenital system

- Micturition pattern D/N
- Urgency
- Urge Incontinence, Stress Incontinence
- Hesitancy
- Stream, continuous, intermittent, double micturition
- Dysuria

I take a detailed micturition pattern history and enquire about urgency, urge, and stress incontinence. Some doctors become rather coy when asking about incontinence. I ask such confronting and indelicate questions as 'do you wet yourself before you can get to the toilet?'

This is one area where the use of plain language, e.g. 'piss, leak' is critical. Coy questions such as, 'Do you have any bladder troubles?' have a much lower yield than, 'Do you ever wet yourself?' It is not the words that matter, it is how you use them. With the right manner, any question can be asked without causing embarrassment to either party.

With men, in addition I enquire about hesitancy, the strength and continuity of the stream, and double micturition. I have numerous diagnoses of prostatic obstruction to my credit and the detection of several neoplasms.

Urinary incontinence is common, and I am often the first practitioner to identify it as a problem. It goes unreported because it has been present for so long that the patient no longer construes it as a problem, for many reasons, including the belief that it is inevitable for someone of their age, and that the way they currently cope is all that can be done.

- Sexuality

This tends to be the point at which both the patient and the partner (in the interview that follows) bring up issues that fall within this category. Again, plain language and a sympathetic, professional, and non-judgemental manner can take us a long way.

Musculo-skeletal system

- Backache
- Joint pain

- Muscle pain
- Mobility problems

Chronic pain is a common issue for elderly people in all situations. Much of it is of musculoskeletal origin, and it does not take a great deal of time to identify and detail spinal and joint problems. With each complaint of pain, I do a very quick pain history which includes localisation, radiation, if the pain is continuous or intermittent, exacerbating and relieving factors, interference with sleep, mobility, daily chores, and recreational activity. I determine the severity of the pain using a basic visual analogue scale.

The medications used in managing chronic pain often cause or exacerbate cognitive impairment and relatively common causes of delirium.

Mobility is a very significant issue and it is simple and straightforward to identify problems. Again, it is very important to get the patient's perspective on what they believe the causes of mobility problems are in their case.

Mobility and balance problems can be verified quickly and easily using the Get up and Go test, and the Modified Romberg test.

At this point I look for signs of extrapyramidal disease, which is a common finding, of obvious significance.

Central nervous system

- Fits, Faints, and Funny Turns

- Falls

- Fractures

- Other

Under the first heading, 'Fits, Faints, and Funny Turns', I explore episodic unsteadiness. I discovered these words in a paper in the Lancet many, years ago. This is an area where the patient's language to describe unsteadiness from all causes is limited to such words as 'dizziness' and 'giddiness'. A worrying number of practitioners accept these terms at face value, assuming that the patient is describing vertigo. This is then followed by some sort of pharmaco-therapeutic reflex prescription of drugs such as Prochlorperazine. In real life, true vertigo which is characterised by the sensation of rotation (either the patient or the world) is a rare cause of unsteadiness that results in falling. Even in the unreal world of Falls Clinics it is also uncommon.

Far, far, more common is postural hypotension. This is easily clarified by asking the patient to describe what 'giddiness' actually feels like in their head. Many will spontaneously describe a feeling of light-headedness and a sense of an impending fall, without ever describing any sense of rotation or symptoms that are associated with vestibular disease. I regularly then go on to ask, 'If you have been sitting down or lying down for a long time, and you stand up quickly, can that cause your giddiness?' A very high proportion, even patients who are not expected to have this degree of awareness, say that they often sit there, or stand for a while, until they feel steady enough to move off. Confirming postural hypotension is extremely easy. It annoys me that elderly patients in hospitals and residential facilities rarely have their blood pressure measured lying and standing. A periodic sitting only blood pressure is of not the slightest use in this, or any other context. I carry a small electronic wrist sphygmomanometer in my bag, and a postural BP drop is easily demonstrated. Prochlorperazine is more often the cause than a cure.

Obviously, falls are an extremely important problem in this patient population. Falls have causes that must be identified and explored. The falls history begins with the question, 'Have you ever fallen over'. Here again the interpretation of language can be an issue. Answers such as, 'I've never fallen over, but I have tripped over a few times', 'I've never had a real fall...', make it obvious that even here where the word seems perfectly clear, patients make their own interpretations. I explain that, 'A fall is a fall... If you hit the ground unexpectedly, that's a fall'.

I then try to establish how long ago the first fall occurred, and when the most recent fall occurred. I ask the patient to tell me in detail about that fall. Where did it happen? (Outdoors? Indoors? Which room?). What were you doing immediately before the fall? (Lying down? Sitting? Standing? Walking?). Did you have any warning that you were going to fall? Did you lose consciousness? Were you able to stand up immediately afterwards? Did you injure yourself? This is not a complete list of questions as the patient's answers direct the further interrogation. For example, if the patient's past medical history and descriptions of events raises the possibility of a cardiac arrhythmia, a seizure, hypoglycaemia, or transient ischaemic attack, detailed questions follow.

What makes falling a problem is twofold. One of the things that people who have fallen or have even been close to falling have in common is that they are very frightened that they will fall again. This is a very real fear that can lead to severe restrictions of activity that can only aggravate the fall risk. The main problem is fracture. The single highest risk factor for future fractures is previous fracture. The risks of fractures in terms of health, independence, and life itself cannot be exaggerated.

A fracture resulting from a fall is presumptive evidence of osteoporosis, and this must be addressed.

Other systems/symptoms

One of the commonest things that I notice, apart from deafness, is very poor vision. The moment I suspect this, I fish out my little test card, and do a rough visual test. It is quite amazing how many of the people presented to me in all settings are virtually blind, unbeknownst to those around them. I am talking about people who can only read the 6/60 line by holding the card right up to their face with both eyes open while wearing their glasses. It answers a lot of questions about their presentation.

The next section looks at alcohol use and medication.

Alcohol intake

Alcohol use is very common in the Australian population, and abuse is also quite common. It is important to ask about this routinely. Again, we may be hesitant to question someone who could be offended.

Alcohol abuse is often a contributing factor in the development of dementia and may be the main causative factor. Serious alcoholics spend most of their pension income on alcohol and cigarettes, leaving little for other necessities of life. When asking about alcohol intake, we should not accept answers such as, 'I only drink occasionally … I'm only a moderate drinker …'. I always detail and quantify. 'What do you mostly drink (beer, wine, spirits)?' 'How many glasses of wine do you drink in the average day, or the average week?'.' How do you buy your wine (bottles, casks)?' 'What size cask (2L,4L, 5L)?' How long does a cask last?). Casks of fortified wine, such as port, are the cheapest sources of high percentage of alcohol. Students have been stunned by the answers.

Late onset alcoholism is not common but can be difficult to detect unless it is specifically looked for. I vividly remember the widow of a senior clergyman who had been almost teetotal for most of her life. I had been asked to see her because of deterioration in her behaviour and self-care and concerns about her safety and ability to continue living in an Independent Living Unit. I arrived at her front door at the same time as she was returning from shopping. I took the shopping bag from her while she opened the door. It contained two bottles of sherry. I learnt that the death of her husband had hit her very hard and having no one to confide in she found solace in alcohol. Her GP and the management of the facility were amazed. They would never ever have suspected that this was possible. We replaced the sherry with an antidepressant and enrolled her in Day Care at the facility.

Alcohol used to be the only substance regularly abused by my patient population. Given that I am now regularly seeing patients who are my contemporaries and people younger than myself, I am now alert to the possibility of other forms of substance abuse. This is the point at which it would be raised and discussed.

Medication

I always ask patients to show me everything that they are taking, prescribed as well as OTC. This is often an interesting exercise. For example, a patient who swears to complete compliance cannot find his medication. Things are written on packets that have no correlation with the contents, e.g. 'For Headache', on a packet of a hypotensive agent, 'Dizziness' on a container of warfarin. A quick look at the dates of when the drug was dispensed compared to the contents is often enlightening.

In a small review of my records, less than 20% of my patients could give a reasonably accurate drug history. This is associated with their cognitive state, but many cognitively intact people also have very little understanding of why they are taking medication, although the majority claim to be taking the medication as prescribed. The implications for compliance are very obvious. We should think seriously about the probability of compliance before reaching for the prescription pad.

Herbal and other 'natural' remedies are used very widely. In fact, they are almost universal. I will discuss this in some detail in a later section, but it is important that their use is considered in the context of medication, as they are not all inert, innocuous, harmless, and free from side-effects and drug interactions.

Psychiatric and social inquiry

This is structured to begin with a quick general psychiatric history. As with the Somatic Inquiry, each item can be expanded as needed.

Appearance/Behaviour

I note and comment on the patient's overall appearance, their alertness and concentration, their affect, and level of anxiety.

Rapport/Conversation

I note how easily the patient is engaged and rapport is achieved, after overcoming the initial hostility and suspicion. I observe the manner of speaking and the use of language, and any elements of dysphasia.

Personality traits

Many of the people that I see have frontal lobe damage, and their apparent personality reflects this.

Sleep pattern

I take a full sleep history, including initial insomnia, broken sleep and it's reasons, resumption after micturition, and early waking.

Energy levels

Energy on waking, energy through the day, day-time napping. Occasionally, the patient makes observations that suggest Sleep Apnoea and I later take this up with a relative.

Depression

In the context of dementia depression is of critical importance. It may invalidate the diagnosis, it may be a comorbidity, and it may be responsible for many of the manifestations that are attributed to dementia alone. I therefore take a full narrative history.

I ask about feelings of depression. This must often be asked in different ways. A lot of elderly people deny depression, with comments such as, 'I would never allow myself to ...', even though everything else they say supports the diagnosis. Many of them object to the word itself, and its connotations. I have had some learned debates on this subject with some of the more pedantic patients. Some say, 'I get a bit down when I'm lonely'. These may be people who have been recently bereaved, and sometimes people who have been bereaved for a long time, but talk as if the death of their spouse was a recent event. Some rationalise their feelings with, 'Of course I'm depressed, the doctor took away my driving licence for no reason'. It must not be forgotten that they are describing a very significant loss, often against background of several losses in succession.

I follow whatever path the patient has gone down. In relatively recent years these travels have taught me how common Post-Traumatic Stress Disorder is in this age group. Incredible events of abuse, including sexual abuse by close relatives, or wartime atrocities ('Dad had been in the German army, but he never said anything about it until now') that had never been spoken of before they suddenly emerge in late life.

Hopelessness. I explore the patient's sense of hopelessness and ask if they have ever felt so low that they wondered if their life was no longer worth living, and if they would be better off dead. It is surprising how many people heartily agree with these sentiments, even many who don't, on the face of it, seem to be particularly depressed. I then ask if they have ever thought of doing away with themselves. If they have, I ask them what they had thought of doing. Medication, firearms, and cars feature prominently in the methodology.

For many, their religious persuasion prevents them from thinking along these lines, but they may add, 'I pray to God every night, asking him to take me away'. One angry old man I saw blamed God for his predicament and the way that he was feeling, and also for refusing to take responsibility by taking him away.

Depressive delusions. I ask about feelings of guilt, worthlessness, et cetera.

Concentration/Interests/Enjoyment. I ask the patient how he likes to fill his time, what interests him, and what he enjoys. I ask about hobbies and social activity. Do you have any regular outings? Do you belong to any groups, organisations, or a church? This tells me a great deal about the depressed patient, who may say that, at this time there is nothing that interests him or that he enjoys.

It also tells me a lot about the person with dementia, who talks about, 'I used to do a lot of …', and describes a progressive shedding of interests, activities, and socialisation.

Anxiety/Panic/Phobias. A lot of my patients describe feelings of apprehension when faced with new social situations and appointments that are sufficient to cause them to panic and avoid virtually all social contact. I have been told many times that people referred to me have been extremely anxious ever since the appointment had been made and had no sleep on the preceding night. When the appointments are being made, I now advise families not to talk about it until the last minute. They often assume that because the patient was present when the referral was discussed with the general practitioner, that there is no reason for the anxiety to manifest.

Delusions and hallucinations. While the delusions are relatively common, it is unusual for patients to complain of them of them or admit to them at this point. One exemption is patients with a paranoid psychosis, which in the British literature used to be described as Senile Paraphrenia. They begin to talk about their delusions from the very outset and are quite preoccupied by them throughout the interview.

Family and social history/relationships

I do a *Family history* (partner, siblings, and children), to identify significant health trends and the diagnosis of dementia.

I take a quick *Biographical history*. Where were you born? Where did you go to school? How many years did you spend at school? Did you complete primary school, did you go on to high school, did you have a tertiary education? What was your work/career after you left school? When were you married? When did you retire? Why did you retire?

With migrants, and I see a great many of these, I ask when did you come to Australia? Did you come by sea? (Most of the people that I see did.) What was the name of the ship? At which port did you disembark? Which migrant hostel did you go to after that? When and how did you end up at (this town)? These are all things that a person who has experienced them as an older child or an adult is very unlikely to forget.

It is important to know the educational history in order to use screening and other tests in a meaningful and valid way. Illiteracy is not rare. I have met several people who have been very successful in life without ever having learnt to read and write more than their signature. They become so skilled at covering up that doctors doing cognitive tests believe that their difficulties writing a sentence is due to a new cognitive impairment.

Marital history. Are you married? The fact that they had been brought to see me by their spouse does not necessarily mean that they will have an accurate understanding of their marital status. A number of delusional beliefs may come to light at this point. What is the first name of your spouse? Are you widowed? How long have you been widowed? How did your spouse die?

Have you had any children? Tell me their names starting with the eldest? Where does (name) live? Do you keep in touch your children? Which of them do you see most of? Again, quite surprising responses may appear.

Other observations/key events/stressors

The referral is often triggered by behavioural changes that have followed a significant event. For example, I recently saw an elderly man with a previous diagnosis of 'mild dementia' who became unsettled, confused, preoccupied, and unable to do and enjoy the things that he and his wife both used to find pleasurable (they played golf and regularly ate out with friends). They had been referred to me by their new general practitioner after they had moved into suburban Adelaide to be near two of their children and grandchildren. At my interview with him, he confided in me that although he and his wife had discussed the pros and cons of moving to Adelaide, and he had agreed that the move made good sense, he nevertheless had not really wanted to move, and now had many regrets that he could not shake off. His wife was quite surprised, because he loved his children and particularly his grandchildren, and she had been convinced that the decision to move had been mutual and that he had been looking forward to it is much as she had.

Living arrangements/ADL/IADL

Type and address of current accommodation. How long have you been living there? Where were you living before that? Living alone, or living with spouse/partner/child/etc.

The fact that dementia is an extremely disabling condition is very poorly appreciated and understood even by practitioners who consider themselves experts in dementia. It is very difficult for people to understand that someone who has minimal visible physical disability, who walks, talks, and seems perfectly capable, can nevertheless be severely disabled.

We measure disability in terms of the Activities of Daily Living. I have strong opinions on the use of instruments in the diagnosis of dementia that I will expand upon in a later section. I do an ADL and an IADL questionnaire made up of lists of common everyday activities and I score them. This is discussed fully later in the chapter when screening instruments are examined.

For scoring purposes, the questionnaire is divided into the patient's *perceptions* (Pt.) and the partner/relative/key carer's *observations* (Carer) which I learn in the course of the Informant Interview. There is often a striking discrepancy between these perceptions and observations that can be seen at a glance.

Each of the IADL items needs to be expanded and detailed. For example, how do you get your meals? Do you cook all your meals? What sort of things do you cook? Meals on Wheels are only delivered five days a week, how do you manage on weekends?

Even people who have previously denied that they are on any medication tend to claim that they are fully compliant.

For very many people driving is much more than just transportation. In answer to the question, 'Do you drive?' it is common to be told, 'If you take my licence away I might as well be dead'.

I ask everyone about their income and how it is managed. If this is likely to be an issue that may call for some form of intervention, I do a more comprehensive financial inquiry that includes greater detail about income and assets, and debts and financial obligations as a preview to a more formal assessment (as discussed under Ethical Issues).

I ask about future plans regarding changes of accommodation and Advance Directives. This is often of immediate relevance in the situation.

When I interview a partner/relative/carer I use the logic of the logic of the Disability Assessment for Dementia (DAD) Test, when examining each item. The test examines each item in terms of executive functions, summarised as Initiation, Planning and Organisation, and Effective Performance. For me this is the most meaningful executive function test, as it addresses the main cause of disability in dementias of all types.

Screening and assessment instruments in suspected dementia

I do all of my testing on completion of the ADL/IADL interview. By then I have achieved the best rapport that I am likely to achieve, and have demonstrated that my interest goes beyond placement, driving, or proving that she is mad for the benefit of all those conspiring against her. I emphasise (yet again) that she is not being singled out, and that what I am doing is routine and applied equally to everybody. I add that she will need to be patient with me if some of the questions seem silly, self-evident, or childish. A common observation is, 'I haven't done anything like that since I was at school, and that was a long time ago'.

What can instruments do?

- Screen: reveal a possible problem/issue
- Facilitate rapid assessment
- Assist in diagnosis
    - Underlying disease process
    - Disability and handicap
    - Social impact
- Quantify to enable evaluation of
    - Severity
    - Progression
- Effects of intervention (Monitoring)
- Allow clear communication (the 'lingua franca')

What do we need instruments to do?

To date, there are no readily available simple and conclusive markers of the disease that can be used to make a firm diagnosis by means of imaging or laboratory testing and the diagnosis is made clinically assisted by a variety of instruments to demonstrate and clarify the various manifestations.

It is in fact unlikely that any simple marker will ever supplant clinical diagnosis because of the diversity of the domains that must be addressed.

The domains that should be addressed include:

- Cognition

Several cognitive domains are commonly impaired in dementia of whatever aetiology – memory, language (communication and comprehension), perceptual skills, attention and concentration, constructive abilities, orientation, calculation, problem solving and functional abilities.

Executive function

- Affect
- BPSD
- Function/Independence
- Decision-making capacity
- Social Impact

I highlight this because I believe that loss of capability with executive function is the critical determinant of the impact of dementia. It explains much of the disability that we see, yet its impact is poorly recognised, poorly understood, and its importance is underestimated. With our obsessive drive to reach a neat diagnosis, it is widely accepted (and expected) that impaired executive function is a major manifestation of some variants of FTD. It is forgotten that it is common in all forms of dementia and almost universal at some point in AD.

Psychologists use the concept to describe a collection of brain processes that control other cognitive processes that are responsible for planning, cognitive flexibility, abstract thinking, rule acquisition, initiation of appropriate actions and inhibition of inappropriate actions, including suppression of automatic responses as well as selection of relevant sensory information. It is generally believed that this system is localised in the prefrontal cortex, although there is some dissention from this view.

For practical purposes, when I teach or explain to relatives, I divide frontal lobe dysfunction into two categories, Personality and Behavioural (see in Informant Interview below), and Intellectual and Dysexecutive.

Intellectual and dysexecutive

- Poor planning and organisational skills;

- Inability to plan and follow through a course of action, and/or

- Failure to complete assignments.

- Impaired judgement;

- Inability to take probable consequences of an action into account;

- Inability to learn from errors;

- Impaired problem-solving skills;

- Loss of capacity to think in abstract terms, inflexibility;

- Impairment of recent memory;

- Reduction in spontaneous speech;

- Word-finding problems, naming problems;

- Perseveration;

- Stereotypic fillers, circumlocution, empty speech.

For me this is what our frontal lobe tests must reveal, and (as I explain below) I do not find the Frontal Assessment Battery particularly useful (or user-friendly) in this regard, and I deduce problems in executive function in other, more meaningful ways.

Design and qualities of tests

Most of the tests that we use in this context were originally designed as research tools and have then been adopted as day-to-day clinical tools. The research approach is of necessity much more rigorous than the workaday clinical approach.

Broadly speaking, different diagnostic tests for the same disease may have different sensitivity and specificity or vice versa:

Sensitivity is defined as the probability of testing positive if the condition is actually present. In general, the more sensitive a test is for a disease, the lower the false negative rate (result negative, but condition present) and the higher the false-positive rate (result positive, but condition absent). This makes a highly sensitive test ideal as a screening examination.

Specificity is defined as the probability of screening negative if the disease is truly absent. The test will rarely be positive in the absence of the condition. Highly specific tests are best in a confirmatory role.

Most of the tests that we use, and the way we use them are screening tests and lack the specificity to be truly diagnostic.

In considering these points, we must realise that there is an underlying assumption that the condition that is in question is a clearly defined entity. While this can almost be assured in the research arena if we accept the diagnostic criteria as laid down in such an authoritative publication such as DSM-5 or ICD-10 as valid, it cannot be guaranteed in what I shall deliberately continue to call the clinical real world.

Another very important characteristic that it is generally taken for granted is that there is inter-rater reliability. This is the degree of agreement among different raters. Outside the research arena, inter-rater reliability is likely to be low. For this, and other reasons that will be discussed, I believe that the clinician should always do his own testing.

It is important to be aware that many factors other than true cognitive impairment can affect test scores. These include:

- Education level
- Cultural & linguistic factors
- Sensory impairment
- Anxiety & depression
- Adverse effects of medication

Cognitive testing

What is always important to remember is that the focus is on an acquired disorder, where there is change from a previous level of functioning in one or more domains.

There are many situations where cognitive testing by an ordinary clinician is simply impossible. Neuropsychologists can do it, but I cannot. That does not preclude me from diagnosing dementia in patients with Down Syndrome, other forms of Intellectual Disability, outback dwelling Aborigines where the living environment is completely foreign to me and language may be an additional issue, or people with whom no useful communication can be established. The diagnosis can be confidently inferred based on the observations of change in cognitive attributes, independent functioning, performance of previously skilled activities, and behaviour, *by people who have known the patient well over a long period of time.*

I use the Montréal Cognitive Assessment (MOCA test) routinely because I find it to be a useful and reliable test that more closely parallels what I have learnt and deduced clinically. I use the MMSE only if I must because it is linked to what can be prescribed under the Pharmaceutical Benefits Scheme in Australia.

Mini Mental State Examination

The MMSE was introduced by Folstein in 1975 and has been extensively researched since that time. Its validity has been confirmed. It is accepted as being a well-documented and validated test that measures cognitive impairment. It is not, as many believe per se diagnostic of AD (Tombaugh and McIntyre), and I question its validity, compared to the modern day clinical assessment based on current understanding of the different cognitive domains.

The MMSE tests a number of domains:

- Orientation
- Registration (memory)
- Attention
- Recall (memory)
- Language
- Verbal fluency (repeat a phrase)
- Nominal aphasia (name 2 objects)
- Receptive aphasia/apraxia (three-stage command)
- Alexia (written command)
- Agraphia (write a sentence)

- Copying (constructional apraxia)

It is not useful for the detection of focal deficits (amnesia, aphasia, visuo-spatial disorders, etc) and is insensitive to frontal lobe disorders. A very major failing is that it does not overtly test executive function.

Administration

The performance and scoring must be done in a rigidly structured and consistent manner. The test is often said to have good inter-rater reliability. This is not strictly correct, as the test is not well standardised despite there being several versions and rules of performance available (see below).

There must not be any coaching or hints, and the interviewer should not indicate in any way that the responses are correct or incorrect. That is not to say that the interviewer should not be reassuring and keep the subject at ease.

I stick to the standardised version developed by Molloy et al. on the rare occasions that I use the instrument and there are very few people whom I trust to do it reliably.

> I am going to ask you some questions and give you some problems to solve. Please try to answer as best you can.
>
> **Orientation in time:** *(Allow 10 seconds for each*

reply. Max 5 points.)

What year is this? *(Accept exact name only.)*

What season is this? *(During the last week of the old season or the first week of the new season accept either answer.)*

What month is this? *(On the first day of the new month or the last day of the old month accept either answer.)*

What is today's date? *(Accept previous or next date.)*

What day of the week is this? *(Accept exact name only.)*

Orientation in place: *(Allow 10 seconds for each reply. From largest to smallest. Max 5 points.)*

What country are we in? *(Accept exact name only.)*

What province/state/county are we in? *(Accept exact name only.)*

What city/town are we in? *(Accept exact name only.)*

(In clinic/hospital) What is the name of this hospital/building? *(Accept exact name only.)*

(In home) What is the street address of this house? *(Accept street name and house number or*

equivalent in rural area.)

(In clinic/hospital) What floor of the building are we on? *(Accept exact name only.)*

(In home) What room are we in? *(Accept exact answer only.)*

Registration: I am going to name three objects. When I have said all three objects, I want you to repeat them. Remember what they are because I am going to ask you to name them again in a few minutes. *(Say them slowly at approximately 1 second intervals.)*

Please repeat the three items for me.

(Score 1 point for each correct reply on the first attempt. Allow 20 seconds for reply. If subject does not repeat all three, repeat until they are learned, or up to 3 times. Max 3 points.)

Attention and calculation: Spell the word WORLD. *(You may help the subject to spell world correctly.)*

Say: Now spell it backwards please. *(Allow 30 seconds to spell backwards. If the subject cannot spell WORLD even with assistance score 0. Max 5 points.)*

Recall: What were the three objects that I asked you to remember? *(Score 1 point for each correct response regardless of the order. Allow 10 seconds. Max 3 points.)*

Language: Show wrist watch. *(Ask: what is this called? Accept 'wristwatch' or 'watch'. Do not accept 'clock', 'time', etc. Allow 10 seconds. Score 1 point for correct response. Max 1 point.)*

Language: Show pencil. *(Ask: what is this called? Accept 'pencil' only. Do not accept 'pen'. Score 1 point for correct response. Max 1 point.)*

Language: I'd like you to repeat a phrase after me: 'no ifs, ands' or buts'. *(Allow 10 seconds for response. Must be exact. Score 1 point for correct repetition. Max 1 point.)*

Language: Read the words on this page and then do what it says. *(Hand the subject the laminated sheet with 'CLOSE YOUR EYES' on it. If the subject just reads but does not then close eyes – you may repeat: read the words on this page and do what it says to a maximum of three times. Allow 10 seconds, score 1 point only if subject closes eyes. Subject does not have to read out loud. Max 1 point.)*

Language: Ask if the subject is right or left handed. Alternate right/left in the statement, e.g. if the subject is right handed say: Take the paper in your left hand ... Take a piece of paper – hold it up in front of the subject and say the following:

Take this paper in your right/left hand; fold the paper in half once, with both hands, and put the paper down on the floor.

(Allow 30 seconds. Score 1 point for each instruction correctly executed. Max 3 points.)

Language: Hand the subject a pencil and paper. Write any complete sentence on this piece of paper. *(The sentence should make sense and involve a subject, verb, and object. Allow 30 seconds. Score 1 point. Max 1 point.)*

Praxis: Place design, pencil and eraser and paper in front of the subject. Say: copy this design please. *(Allow multiple tries until the subject is finished and hands it back. Maximum time 1 minute. The subject must have drawn a four-sided figure between two five-sided figures. Score 1 point for correctly copied diagram. Max 1 point.)*

Interpretation

In this, and other screening tests, it is useful to think of the performance and the interpretation as separate steps to avoid attempting to influence the performance to achieve a pre-conceived required score or any other reason. Folstein himself argued this.

I believe that the way the patient performs the test is almost as important as the score. I jot down shorthand observations as the test proceeds. Examples include 'Tense and anxious +++'; 'Distractible +++', 'Rationalisations ++-' and long explanations why some items of information are not needed by the patient, e.g. 'I don't need to remember the address because …', 'Very slow to initiate'. I write down the patient's exact responses, for example, under the date I write the actual answer, 29th. While one of the main criticisms of the MMSE is that it does not test executive function, there can be many clues observed and noted in the way that the patient performs – 'Unable to initiate, 'very slow', 'disorganised method'.

Normal elderly persons score an average of 27.6. A score of 24–30 suggests no cognitive impairment, 20–23 mild, and 10–19 moderate, and 0–9 severe impairment. In established dementia, the MMSE score deteriorates by about 4 points per year. A simple way of interpreting the score is: below 24, probable cognitive impairment; below

17, definite cognitive impairment.

Increasingly, a score below 26 is seen as a good trade-off between sensitivity and specificity. In short, patients like this should be reviewed periodically.

There are ceiling effects. Cognitively adept people may have a significant cognitive deficit affecting ability and behaviour, but still perform well on the MMSE.

There is also a floor effect. Progression cannot be assessed beyond the point when the severely demented patient can score only a few points. I do not have a problem with this as my assessment of severity progression is clinically based.

In normal and demented subjects, most of the errors occurred in recall of the three words, attention and concentration, copying the pentagons, and orientation in time.

The MMSE performance is affected by

- age,
- pre-morbid intelligence,
- language,
- education, and
- socio-economic status, as well as by
- psychiatric illness and

- somatic illness-related factors such as
  - depression,
  - delirium,
  - conditions affecting concentration, motivation,
- medication.

I believe that the MMSE has become dangerously misleading and should be abandoned. A very large number of general practitioners and a good many specialists in relevant fields rely on the MMSE score as *absolute evidence of the presence or absence of dementia*, 'A score of 24–30 suggests no cognitive impairment …'. This often becomes a reason for failure to refer, even when partners and relatives express their concerns about someone's actual real-life cognitive performance.

As an assessment of severity, 'A score of 24–30 suggests no cognitive impairment, 20–23 mild, and 10–19 moderate, and 0–9 severe impairment.' Anyone with any serious experience of dementia assessment will have confidently and accurately diagnosed dementia in many people with scores within the 'no cognitive impairment' range.

What is much more concerning is that many, including leading specialists in this field date the onset of dementia from the transition of the MMSE score below 24/30. It is staggering that any intelligent person, let alone a specialist in this field can seriously believe this to be the fact.

What does severity mean? Is it a measure of the impact of the sum of the cognitive impairments, changes in behaviour, capacity for independent function, changes in personality? Does it mean the stress and burden faced the partner, and the risk of breakdown of the relationship? There is no screening test that measures all of this. There are tests that deal with some aspects, but we should conduct structured face-to-face interviews that can explore relevant issues in depth, not look for some new no-touch technique that can justify yet another survey.

Severity rated by MMSE score is useless.

The Montreal Cognitive Assessment

As noted above, I now use the MOCA as my routine screening test. I used to use the ADAS-Cog for testing high MMSE scorers, which was allowed by the PBS (surely an admission of the fallibility of the MMSE). It was designed to screen for Mild Cognitive Impairment. It was introduced in 2005. As a sample of segments of more comprehensive neuropsychological assessments it is a considerably better sample, that does not include the 'freebies' that guarantee easy points on the MMSE (e.g. immediately repeating three words).

It covers a number of domains including:

- concentration, attention (digit repetition, random letter test);
- orientation (recent memory);
- new learning ability;
- short-term memory, immediate recall;
- language
    - naming,
    - similarities, abstraction (conceptualisation, logical thinking),
    - words in 1 minute (lexical fluency, mental flexibility);
- visuo-constructional skills;
- visual-motor sequencing;
- executive function (the MOCA includes a a trail test and a version of a clock drawing test).

Using a cut-off score of 26, the MMSE had a sensitivity of 18% compared to the MOCA's 90% in detecting MCI subjects. For mild Alzheimer's disease, the sensitivity was 78% for the MMSE, and 100% for the MOCA. Specificity was high with both.

For a time, I did both the MMSE and the MOCA on all patients. I have many, many examples of people who scored in the high 20s on the MMSE, scored in the high teens on the MOCA. In all of these cases, the MOCA correlated much more closely with what I had concluded clinically.

Clock drawing

Clock drawing requires a number of cognitive skills, a mix of visuospatial abilities and executive control functions (Shulman K, Feinstein A), including:

1. Comprehension (auditory)
2. Planning
3. Visual memory and reconstruction in a graphic image
4. Visuospatial abilities
5. Motor programming and execution
6. Numerical knowledge
7. Abstract thinking (semantic instruction)
8. Inhibition of the tendency to be pulled by perceptual features of the stimulus (i.e. the 'frontal pull' of the hands to '10' in the

instruction 'ten past eleven')

9.   Concentration and frustration tolerance

There are numerous versions, but I believe that the CLOX version (Royall) gives me the most information about executive function.

The test is in two parts:

CLOX 1: The patient is presented with a blank sheet of paper and instructed to 'draw a clock that shows 1:45 and set the hands and numbers on the face so that even a child could read them'. The instructions can be repeated until understood, but no further guidance is given after the task has commenced.

The official form has a printed circle that is visible through the paper in the lower left-hand corner.

This requires the patient choose the clock's overall form (analog or digital face etc) shape, size, position on the paper, and the elements (numbers, hands), and avoid the distraction of the circle that is visible. The words 'face' and 'hands' are deliberately chosen because they represent parts of the body.

CLOX 2: The patient watches the examiner draw a clock in the prepared circle and is then asked to copy it.

Scoring:

Organisational Elements Points CLOX 1 CLOX 2

Does figure resemble a clock? 1

Outer circle present? 1

Diameter> 1 inch? 1

All numbers inside the Circle? 1

12, 6, 3, & 9 placed first? 1

Spacing intact? 2

If spacing errors are present,

are there signs of correction or erasure 1

Only Arabic numerals? 1

Only numbers 1-12 among

the Arabic numerals present? 1

Sequence 1-12 intact?

No omissions or intrusions 1

Only two hands present? 1

All hands represented as arrows? 1

Hour hand between 1 and 2 o'clock? 1

Minute hand longer than hour hand? 1

None of the following:

(1) hand pointing to 4 or 5 o'clock

(2) '1-45' present

(3) intrusions from hand or face present

(4) any letters words or pictures

(5) any intrusion from circle below

I must confess that I only rarely do the test so rigorously, but, as with all tests I learn from the principles, and the logic behind the test, rather than becoming obsessed with the significance of a precise score.

Frontal Assessment Battery

I have another confession to make. I no longer do the FAB, and I do not miss it. I strongly believe that a test should reveal something that can increase my understanding of what I am faced with. If I cannot fully understand how a test or an item explains an important manifestation, and cannot convey that understanding to a patient, and more importantly a partner/relative or key carer, then it is of little use to me, or anybody else.

I do not need a test instrument to diagnose impaired executive function any more than I need one to diagnose depression or anxiety. These are fundamentally clinical diagnoses, and if a test does not confirm my clinical diagnosis, then I am confident enough to conclude that the test is misleading and I can often see how a misleading test result has been achieved.

That is a long preamble to my confession that I don't know how to use the FAB to explain why mother can no longer bake the cakes that she had once been famous for. A score of 9/18 means nothing to me, and even less to that relative. I can use the outcome of a clock drawing test to explain mother's growing difficulty in baking her cake or undertaking any ADL or IADL activity, particularly if I use the logic of the DAD in my explanation.

Neuropsychological assessment

I am a great admirer of neuropsychology, and the huge advances that neuropsychological research has made in our understanding of cognitive disorders. I have worked closely with several neuropsychologists over the years and have learnt a great deal from them.

In most cases, I would rather have a neuropsychologist's opinion than an MRI. However, I find that neuropsychologists who have worked predominantly in a Memory Clinic setting, even though they bear the title of Clinical Neuropsychologist, may be more scientist than clinician.

Many of the tests conducted by neuropsychologists are somewhat abstract, and, even more than the FAB, difficult to translate into everyday reality. What results in the report may then be very inconclusive.

A report I received on testing executive function

read as follows, 'Whilst his copy of a complex geometrical figures showed some poor planning, the final product was soundly within age-based expectation. Cognitive flexibility was again severely impaired. Ability to shift mental set on a simple sorting task was similarly impaired. Although he was able to form a simple concept, he was unable to shift mental set, and his performance was characterised by some concrete and inflexible thinking'. On clinical examination, comparing his perception with the observations of his partner and family, there is no question that he meets all the criteria of executive dysfunction.

This report is undergraduate. It is not what I would have received from the experienced neuropsychologists that I have worked with, consulted, or reviewed in medicolegal situations. They would all have been aware that very important decisions would be influenced by their opinions. I say opinions, because raw data is meaningless in this context, and this context must be understood. The data must be expertly interpreted. This requires understanding of the context and the real-life implications of the cognitive failings that are revealed. In other words, the science must be interpreted, and that this interpretation is moulded by reasoning and experience that goes beyond the capacity to elicit findings. This is the art that complements the science. This applies to every discipline that makes up a multidisciplinary team that is assembled in a Memory Clinic.

Psychological tests, tests in BPSD

This is a very important domain for testing. It is devastating when the presence of the conditions that they uncover is missed completely or underestimated.

Anxiety and depression

Anxiety and depression are extremely common co-morbidities in dementia and can also affect performance on cognitive and other testing. They also commonly co-exist. There are numerous available instruments in this area. Again, it must be remembered that they are screening instruments that alert us to the need to undertake a further assessment, and that they cover issues that are included in the diagnostic criteria for the condition.

DSM-IV Criteria for depression (I am aware of DSM-V, but it does not alter the essence of what I am saying):

A patient must exhibit either of the following symptoms almost daily for a 2-week period:

- Depressed mood;
- Markedly diminished interest or pleasure in usually pleasurable activities *plus* any four of the following:
  - Significant weight loss or, atypically, weight gain;

- Insomnia or hypersomnia;

- Psychomotor agitation or retardation;

- Fatigue or loss of energy;

- Feelings of worthlessness or excessive inappropriate guilt;

- Diminished ability to think or to concentrate, indecisiveness;

- Recurrent thoughts of death, suicidal ideation, suicide attempt, or a specific plan for suicide.

By far the commonest instrument used internationally is the Geriatric Depression Scale (GDS). It has a high sensitivity and specificity. It was originally a 30-point questionnaire. This was reduced to 15 items with no loss of specificity or sensitivity and is commonly used in this form.

Geriatric Depression Rating Scale (short form)

Are you basically satisfied with your life?

Have you dropped many of your activities and interests?

Do you feel that your life is empty?

Do you often get bored?

Are you in good spirits most of the time?

Are you afraid that something bad is going to happen to you?

Do you feel happy most of the time?

Do you often feel helpless?

Do you prefer to stay at home, rather than going out and doing new things?

Do you feel you have more problems with memory than most?

Do you think it is wonderful to be alive now?

Do you feel pretty worthless the way you are now?

Do you feel full of energy?

Do you feel that your situation is hopeless?

Do you think that most people are better off than you?

Questions are scored Yes/No. Cut-off normal range is 0–5, above 5 suggests depression.

1 Yes / 2 Yes / 3 Yes / 4 Yes / 5 No / 6 Yes / 7 No / 8 Yes / 9 Yes / 10 Yes / 11 No / 12 Yes / 13 No / 14 Yes / 15 Yes

There is an even shorter form (5 questions):

1. Are you basically satisfied with your life? *(No)*

2. Do you often get bored? *(Yes)*

3. Do you often feel helpless? *(Yes)*

4. Do you prefer to stay at home rather than going out and doing new things? *(Yes)*

5. Do you feel pretty worthless the way you are now? *(Yes)*

I take a psychiatric history, so I rarely use instruments, but there are times when communication is so difficult I look to the tests for inspiration for something to ask and talk about.

The Cornell Scale for Depression in Dementia is widely used in the residential sector in Australia. It covers the important vegetative signs of dementia much better than the GDS, and again I use items from it in my psychiatric inquiry.

The Montgomery and Asberg Depression Rating Scale is a very good scale to explore the feelings of more cognitively intact patients.

I rarely rely on screening tests. I prefer to do a structured interview using items common to most of the tests and the diagnostic criteria from DSM-5. The patient's understanding of terms can be determined, and allowances made. Any point can be explored more fully and different tracks pursued without constraint. The patient's emotional responses can be clearly seen. I do not base my diagnostic judgements on test scores, but on my clinical impression.

Function

This is measured by the patient's ability to perform the Basic Activities of Daily Living (ADLs) and the Instrumental Activities of Daily Living (IADLs). Again, there are numerous scales.

The Barthel Index is one of the oldest ADL indexes used in Geriatrics and Rehabilitation. I use a simplified version that I score from the patient's perceptions. I later score the observations of a partner/relative/carer. This often demonstrates the unawareness of the patient of her situation, needs, and capabilities.

For IADL screening, I use a simplified version of the Lawton IADL scale. It too is one of the oldest tests in the business.

Basic Activities of Daily Living

ADL	ADL Scoring	
• Bathing	• Unable to perform task	1
• Grooming	• Very dependent &/or maximal assistance	2
• Feeding, Eating		
• Toilet Use	• Moderate assistance or supervision	3
• Dressing	• Minimal assistance or supervision	4
• Transfers		
• Walking	• Independent	5
• Wheel Chair Use		
• Stairs		

Instrumental Activities of Daily Living

IADL	IADL Scoring	
• Meal Preparation	2	Independent
• Shopping	1	Assisted
• Housework	0	Dependent
• Laundry		
• Medication Management		
• Telephone		
• Travel		
• Finance		

When quizzing the relative/carer, I explore the details using the logic of the Disability Assessment for Dementia (DAD) that I have already waxed eloquent about, because for me it is everything that a test should be.

Disability Assessment for Dementia (DAD) Scale

- Three components:
  - Basic ADLs
  - Instrumental ADLs
  - Leisure and Housework Activities
- Each activity is divided into three elements:
  - Initiation (goal selection)
  - Planning and Organisation
  - Effective Performance

On the completion of the cognitive testing, I end the patient interview with words such as, 'Well that's it. That's all we need to do. That wasn't too scary, was it? … Tell you what though, as you obviously noticed, there are few holes in your memory. We should be able to help with that, but I need to get a bit more information from your daughter. Is it okay with you if I have a chat with her by herself?' I then lead the patient back to the waiting room and invite the relative(s) to come into the consulting area.

As I have mentioned previously, I try to make sure that there is someone who can entertain and distract the patient while the partner, relatives, and key carers are being interviewed. This is not always easy, and every alternative may need to be explored. When I see people in my rooms, it is my wife. When I am working with a Social Worker, we alternate. At Rural Community Health Centres, the desk staff, who are all local people can assist, although their ability to chase escapees is somewhat limited. Sometimes, the family group is quite large, and the one least up to date on what is happening to the patient, such as a grandchild of any age can be enlisted. The Social Worker learns a lot on this contact, and my wife also learns useful information about the patient's concerns and fears and family dynamics.

Depending on the situation, I may bring the patient back to the consulting room for a summation after interviewing the partner/relatives and key carers.

Informant interview

The informant interview is a critical step in the initial assessment of every patient in every setting. It is particularly important when we are dealing with a resident in an aged care facility. The commonest reason for which I am asked for advice is when there are unresolved behavioural issues complicating the management of the resident. Most of these residents have been diagnosed with dementia at some point. Most do not have the capacity to make rational decisions regarding their health, safety, welfare, or the management of their affairs, and there is someone who has been chosen by them or a legal tribunal to be the substitute decision-maker. Most often this is a close relative. While this is the legal reality, it is not always well understood by those caring for the afflicted person in various capacities. I regularly become aware of tensions and grievances on the part of the relatives based on poor understanding and poor communication. This is a very important part of the background and the context of the behavioural disturbance and its management.

In keeping with my unshakeable belief that dementia affects a relationship, not just an individual, understanding the effect on the partner is as important as diagnosing the afflicted one. The relationship continues to be a central concern, irrespective of the current living arrangements.

I regularly refer partners and relatives to their general practitioners for investigation and management of very diagnosable and treatable conditions.

It is also very important to interview partners/relatives/carers in a structured way. This is a difficult experience for them and they may be very ambivalent about expressing their concerns. In the course of the interview, many relatives become more open and address issues that they would not have thought of without prompting. More, and new information may also come to light during the summation that I describe below.

I begin by explaining that we will go through a detailed structured interview but that I would like them to tell me their most pressing concerns about the patient and the issues in summary.

It often becomes apparent that the partner had to be persuaded by her family to seek a referral for this consultation and is having second thoughts about discussing the situation. She will deny any difficulties, until a daughter or son says, 'Come on mum, you come to me crying every other day, so tell the doctor about it.' At this point, I explain that I need to understand what is happening if I am to be of any help, and only she can tell me what happens when she and her partner are alone together through the day.

It is the partner not the patient who needs support during the interview.

When there is no support of this kind, I still continue with the structured inquiry in detail, and a lot of the reluctant sceptics only begin to voice their concerns during what I call, 'The crash course in dementia' at the end.

Confirmation of history from patient

Where a patient has been very vague about marital status, date of bereavement, how many children there have been, et cetera, I establish the actual details.

Often the conditions uncovered in the somatic inquiry are of major significance and I confirm to what extent they are known to the general practitioner and how they are being managed. Quite often patients who are being treated for pain with opiates have failed to mention it during the inquiry and may even have denied that pain is an issue.

Information Interview

- Identification – Relationshop to patient
- Summary of main concerns
- Confirmation of Medical History, Family History
- Communication – Changes in patient's ability to communicate
- Memory – Observed changes in memory
- Behavioural & Psychiatric Symptoms in Dementia
- Activities/Interests/Social Participation
- ADL/IADL and family expectations & plans

Details of medication use are discussed under the item 'Medication' in the IADL section. (See 'Living Arrangements/ADLs/IADLs' below.)

It is more often the relatives than the patient who report a family history of dementia.

Communication

I often say, 'I noticed that your mother was having great difficulty finding the words for what she wanted to say, have you been noticing this?' If the answer is 'yes', I ask 'when did you first become aware of this?' If the speech pattern is highly suggestive of frontal lobe pathology, we go into details regarding this. In more advanced cases I ask questions about comprehension as well as expression.

Memory

I open by asking, 'When was the very first time that any of you suspected that your mother's memory was less than 100%?' Relatives initially tend to date the first appearance of cognitive problems from some relatively recent event. 'Mum had a pretty good memory until she broke her hip and they gave her an anaesthetic.' Another very common observation is, 'She was all right until dad died, and then she completely fell apart.' The revelation of dementia often follows a significant stressor and when this is pointed out to them partners and relatives begin to understand how stressors cause exacerbations of behavioural and functional problems.

If they do admit that mother's memory has been deteriorating for longer than that, they often qualify it, 'Her memory for what happened in the past is remarkable, much better than mine, but it is recent things that she tends to forget … nothing really important.'

Even more common is, 'It's only her Short-term memory.'

I then go into detail and we cover (with examples), forgetfulness, repetitiveness (one of the issues many carers find particularly difficult to deal with: 'I just told you … You know damned well what day it is!'), losing and misplacing things, forgetting what she has set out to do, forgetting what she has started and not completed before becoming distracted (leaving things on the stove, leaving hoses running, et cetera), forgetting what she has already done (taking her morning medication for the third time). I also ask if she has forgotten how to do things that she used to the able to do really well (e.g. knitting, cooking, using a computer), if can she use all her appliances, and if she can learn to use new appliances (a mobile phone, a microwave, a TV remote control).

During this inquiry, the timescale often shifts quite dramatically, from months to years.

Delusions

Danger, stealing, infidelity, intruders, not home, TV, misidentification

This and following sections are based on the items in the Neuro-psychiatric Inventory (without the rigorous quantification). I ask about each in detail, using common examples.

Danger, threat, suspicion

In this section, the common delusions seen in dementia are confirmed or discovered for the first time. The explanation below is what the patient may have talked about during the interview, and what we are looking for from an observer's perspective.

What I have labelled 'Danger' is a catchall term for beliefs based on fear and suspiciousness that someone wishes them harm and is conspiring against them. Some degree of suspiciousness is almost universal. The question, 'What's all this about?' can recur throughout the interview with the patient. An explanation easily allays it, but it is not easily eliminated. We should be aware, even if we have taken pains to explain that we are not acting on anyone's behalf, and are completely dedicated to the patient's best interest, we are nevertheless likely to be included among the suspected conspirators.

At the other extreme, there is overt paranoia. The inconsistencies illustrate the unreality of delusional thinking inherent in the perception. A woman whose main presenting concerns was, 'It's my daughter. She is trying to run my life. She is always telling me what to do', later went on to proclaim that she did not need any help because she had a wonderful daughter, who did everything for her. *The partner is often the main suspect in this, as in most of the other delusional beliefs.*

The NeuroPsychiatric Inventory

– Input obtained from caregivers or members of the nursing team in the Nursing Home Version

– Structured interview

– Frequency and severity assessed & quantified for

- Delusions
- Hallucinations
- Agitation
- Depression/Dysphoria
- Anxiety
- Euphoria/Elation

- Apathy/Indifference
- Disinhibition
- Irritability/Lability
- Aberrant Motor Behaviour
- Night-time Behaviour
- Appetite/Eating

Stealing

The commonest by far is the belief that anything that she has lost, misplaced, or even hidden, has been taken by 'someone'. These accusations also range from, 'you must have put it somewhere' to the belief that the police must be called. The 'someone' who is accused is often a near relative or carer but can include any recent visitor or a suspected intruder.

Infidelity

The patient believes that when her spouse has gone out for reasons that she has forgotten, that he has been on an assignation. Commonly, a helpful neighbour or family friend is identified as the keeper of the tryst.

I once saw an elderly man who was seriously depressed and delusional, who had been visited by a volunteer who spoke his language. The patient's wife was in the patient's room. The volunteer, who had a fine sense of humour, said to the wife, 'You may as well go out and meet your lover, while we have some man talk.' After this visit, the patient became intensely paranoid and suicidal, asking the nurses to administer an overdose. Needless to say, that volunteer is no longer welcome.

Intruders

The patient believes that someone comes into the home or onto the property, generally to steal things. Sometimes the intruders are more sinisterly threatening, and this causes the patient to become extremely security conscious. Whatever security arrangements are made, they are never sufficient, and need to be replaced.

Sometimes the patient believes that someone else is living in the house and may insist that a place be laid the table, and other provisions be made for that extra person.

Not home

The patient may believe that she lives somewhere else. I have seen patients who have been long term residents in a facility who believe that they are still living with their parents on the family farm. I have seen patients who believe that they still live in a different town, city, or state. This is often somewhere that they had lived in the past.

TV

Sometimes patients identify with events on the television as happening in their lives in the here and now. 'Quick, quick, lock the door. There is a man with a gun outside.' Some enter into conversation with the people on television.

Misidentification

This is the belief that someone is somebody else. It can be very distressing for a spouse or child, when they are not recognised as such. At this point it sometimes also comes to light that she believes that her parents are alive, and talks of other deceased people as if they were still alive.

It is crucial that these delusions be identified, because they have a major impact on the patient's perceptions, behaviour, decision-making, and relationships.

Hallucinations

Visual, auditory, olfactory, tactile, gustatory et cetera. From my observation, vivid hallucinations are a common feature of delirium, although they can be seen in the absence of delirium.

Sometimes the delusions and hallucinations are combined. Intruders may not only be people who are suspected of coming into the home. They may also be people who are visible, with whom they tried to talk, and who may actually be living with them. Sometimes, it is the person that the patient sees in the mirror.

Loss of insight

Very few partners and relatives are aware that the afflicted one has a different perspective on what is happening than they do. I deal with this later (below).

Agitation/Aggression/Resistiveness

This is a very common problem and many partners and relatives complained that, 'Dad's become a different person, he was always a gentle person, but now he's so nasty …'.

One way of looking at agitation is as anxiety, inner turmoil, put into action. Many things can trigger agitation. Some things, such as contradictions, complaints about repetitiveness, strong directions about what to do and how to behave, happen regularly during a day. Agitation leads to anger and aggression, which may be expressed verbally, but may also become physical. Physical aggression is much more common than is suspected, and it often takes a direct question for it to be revealed. In residential facilities, it commonly manifests as resistiveness to needed care.

It is often 'the last straw' for the carer, and a much more compelling trigger for referral for an assessment than functional disability. In its most troublesome presentation, it is as if the patient has acquired an Antisocial Personality Disorder late in life.

Depression/Anxiety

The response to this line of questioning is often surprising. I regularly see patients where their depression is so obvious and so profound that I cut the assessment short, having made the decision that the depression must be addressed urgently, and that a cognitive assessment would be pointless at this time. Whatever the setting, it is not at all unusual for relatives and carers to respond to the question, 'Does your mother seem to be depressed to you?' in the negative. I begin to feel that depression, like myxoedema, is best diagnosed by a stranger. It is not that these relatives and carers are unfeeling, it is just that these conditions evolve slowly and relatives may simply be too close to have observed a difference.

Where depression seems to be a significant issue I enquire about activities, interests, and social participation at this point. I also ask about irritability and explore the vegetative signs of depression including appetite, weight loss, tiredness, and sleep pattern to complete a diagnosis of depression.

Anxiety takes many forms, and I believe that it is pointless trying to separate anxiety from depression in this age group. One very common form of anxiety is seen when the patient becomes anxious and agitated when the spouse is not at home or simply not visible. Again, this ranges from agitation and some argument, 'Where have you been?', to actual searching. The patient will come to the toilet door and knock, 'Are you in there? When are you coming out?' This 'shadowing' is extremely stressful for the carer. It results in the common complaint, 'I can't leave him alone for one minute.'

This is also the point where the family often tells me about previously unknown traumatic events from the patient's past that have emerged as a major 'obsession' and stressor for the patient.

Elation/Euphoria, Apathy/Indifference, Disinhibition, Irritability/Lability

What I label for shorthand as 'Frontal lobe behaviour' includes many things that are perhaps the most difficult and stressful manifestations of dementia that the carer must come to terms with. It is akin to dealing with Mr Hyde, when you are expecting Dr Jekyll. I have had relatives say to me, 'I've lost my mum, she is not there anymore.'

This is a topic that I feel very strongly about and I have preached this message repeatedly. I have listed the behavioural changes in the section dealing with frontal lobe function and will only emphasise a few.

For simplicity, I have itemised the issues that arise from frontal lobe dysfunction into two categories, Personality and Behavioural, and Intellectual and Dysexecutive. I will deal with the latter in this section.

Personality and behavioural issues

- Lack of inhibition
- Impulsivity

- Inappropriate and embarrassing behaviour
- Neglect or unconcern for personal appearance
- Lack of insight
- Lack of concern and empathy for others
- Limited capacity to cope with personal relationships
- Compulsive stealing or hoarding
- Puerile humour, facetiousness
- Mild euphoria, with increased talkativeness and confabulation
- Emotional lability
- Irascibility and verbal aggression
- Striking vulnerability to interference from irrelevant stimuli
- Apathy
- Lack of initiative and spontaneity

The Jekyll and Hyde analogy is appropriate. We are seeing someone whose personality seems to have undergone a permanent dramatic change. This 'other mum' lacks social filters and exhibits many of the above behaviours. She can say very hurtful things without being aware of their impact on the object of her observations. Relatives often believe that they are said with calculated malicious intent.

I once saw an elderly woman with her very supportive daughter on whom she was totally dependent. As the three of us were talking, as an aside, the mother suddenly observed, 'You're just a filthy slut.' The daughter burst into tears. Her mother looked at her in surprise and asked, 'What's the matter with you, it's true, isn't it?' Her 'old mum', would have died rather than said such a thing.

Aberrant motor activity

At this point I focus on restlessness and wandering. In residential care, other types of aberrant motor activity are much more common than in the community dwelling population. However, in the community the consequences may be much more severe when someone wanders off and becomes lost. This can also happen in vehicles.

Sleep/Night-time behaviour

I learn the sleeping pattern from the carer's perspective. Nocturnal disturbance is very common in residents of aged care facilities and is not rare in the home situation either. I vividly recall the problems faced by the wife of a very disturbed man whom we had admitted trying to control his behaviour. She was very determined that she would continue to care for him at home. It was very, very, difficult to manage him even in a secure environment staffed by skilled psychiatric nurses. We held a case conference with her and asked her for her bottom line. What did we have to guarantee before she would take him back home. Her bottom line was, 'I need to have at least one decent night's sleep a week.'

Relatives often describe a sleep pattern very suggestive of Obstructive Sleep Apnoea. It is worth excluding, but few patients with advanced dementia can cope with CPAP.

Appetite/Eating disorder

I have already commented on loss of appetite and weight loss being common problems in dementia. It is important to establish what the appetite is like in every patient and to identify weight loss. Weight loss is an important feature of dementia. There are many causes, one of which, is simply forgetting to eat. Sometimes families assume that delivered meals are being eaten, despite the weight loss of the patient and the growing obesity of her little dog. Executive dysfunction is important to identify as some people with advanced dementia may need prompting to pick up a spoon and eat, even though they are hungry.

Interests and activity

I ask how the patient likes to occupy herself through the day. Handcrafts? TV? Reading? etc. Are there any regular outings? Does she belong to any organisations, clubs, or church?

Where there is a significant cognitive impairment, there is a progressive narrowing of the range of activities and interests eventually ending with 'She doesn't do anything, she just sits in front of the TV.' Sometimes there is a deleterious addition to this, 'He just sits around smoking and drinking beer.'

Driving

Even though this item is included in the IADL assessment, its potentially so traumatic for all concerned, that it warrants special attention.

Like the patients, relatives often express concern with a veiled threat, 'If you take away his licence it will kill him.' I nevertheless go on to ask if they have any concerns about the parent's driving, including accidents and offences. Does he get lost going to familiar places? Does he drive very slowly? When you have travelled with him did he obey all the road rules? Has he had any vehicle accidents or been stopped by the police? Would you let him pick up your children from school?

Advance directives

I ask if these are in place. In South Australia, there are two that are relevant. These are the Enduring Power of Attorney that covers financial issues, and Advanced Care Directive (which replaced the Enduring Power of Guardianship in 2013), which covers both medical and lifestyle decisions. I explain the purpose of these Powers and strongly urge that both be organised as quickly as possible (yesterday).

Living arrangements/ADLs/IADLs

I confirm the actual living arrangements. Patients regularly tell me that they live with their parents on the farm, or they live in another town at a previous address. Bed-fast disabled people who are reduced to living in one room, equipped with a hospital bed and a commode, often tell me these things. Our obsession with keeping people in their home at all costs should be tested by reality from time to time.

We then go through the ADL items in detail. Resistiveness to showering is a very common finding even in people seen as reasonably compliant ('I already had a shower this morning'). Grooming is often a clue when someone who has been very meticulous about her appearance becomes oblivious to it. When she eats, does she use utensils? Do you have to prompt her to begin or to keep eating? Have you observed any difficulties with swallowing? Does she start to cough while she is eating? Does food sometimes come straight back at her?

Dressing problems can also become known, ranging from becoming less meticulous and progressing to complete inability. This is where the logic of the DAD comes into its own. Who decides that it is time to get dressed? Who chooses the clothing? Does she dress in the correct sequence (underwear before top clothes)? Do you have to keep prompting her to continue? If you put a shirt in front of her, would she know what to do with it?

Can she stand and transfer without standby or assistance? Can she walk safely without standby or assistance? Does she move off without her walking aids? Have there been any falls? How many falls have there been in the last six months? Has she ever injured herself in fall? Has she had to be taken to hospital because of a fall?

Each of the IADLs must also be addressed in detail. Where do your mother's meals come from? She says that she cooks all her meals, is that true? How good is her cooking nowadays? Are you sure that she actually eats the Meals on Wheels? Do you look in her fridge from time to time to see if there is food there that is beginning to go off?

What does she buy when she goes shopping? Is she always buying the same things (I call this routine shopping) whether she needs them or not? Is she buying a lot of sweets and biscuits rather than proper food?

How is her housework getting done? A common response is that the family had organised a cleaner, but she was sent away because she was not needed or was too expensive.

Who is doing the laundry? Again, the patient has often claimed that she does all the laundry including the linen, but the family reports that she has forgotten how to use the washing machine. One patient had stopped using washing powder because she deemed it too expensive and unnecessary and her family learnt to spirit away her laundry when she was not looking and return it in pristine condition.

Does she take her medicines regularly? Do you look at the Webster Pak when you visit?

Does she use her telephone correctly? Can she call for assistance if needed? Does she ring you at unreasonable times?

What is her income? (Pension, Superannuation, self-funded retiree, etcetera.) Can she manage her finances? Does she have unpaid bills? Has she been threatened with cessation of services from non-payment? Does she squander her money? Does she gamble on the pokeys? Does she get persuaded to buy things she does not need because of persuasive salespeople or TV ads? Does she make large donations to charity in response to visitors or phone calls? Do you help her to keep her finances in order?

The crash course in dementia: *'What have we learnt?'*

This is the most important thing that I do. I review my findings and what I have learnt from interviewing and examining the patient, and from other sources of information, particularly the partner/relative interview and explain what this reveals about what is happening to the afflicted person and how it impacts upon the partner. I also explain that before I complete my report, I may need to seek further information from doctors and hospitals.

I leave this section till last because in effect this details my conceptualisation of the origins of the major manifestations of dementia and how the disability and behavioural disturbance that results from the pathological damage can be explained by the loss of specific cognitive functions in ways that make sense to me and more importantly to the partner, relatives, and carers. It enables problems to be addressed more objectively and treat the manifestations as common parts of part of the syndrome rather than complications.

This conceptualisation continues to evolve. Teaching, and answering probing questions from intelligent students, partners, and relatives drives me to think, research and study.

The current conventional conceptualisation is ridiculously simplistic. The idea that the be all, and end all, of cognitive impairment is something that can be proved or disproved by a simple memory test should be patently and obviously seen as absurd, yet extremely important decisions are regularly being made by neurologists, psychiatrists, geriatricians, and other specialists on just that inadequate information.

At the outset, I explain that dementia is caused by any disease or injury that extensively damages the brain and destroys brain tissue. Many, but not all, of these causes are progressive. This damage means that the brain does not work as well as it used to and that this causes many losses of functions and abilities that we will now examine in detail.

Memory is about handling information: its acquisition, processing, storing, maintaining, accessing and applying. We use the information from memory continuously. We must be able to make and use new memories until the day we die. They are the building blocks of our all our thoughts and actions. When we want that specific memory, we recall it, usually by remembering it, and there it is. However, when the brain is damaged this system can fail at any point.

A piece of information is anything that we receive through our senses. By far the most important information that we receive consciously is through communication with language. If there are difficulties in the reception, interpretation and the processing of language, this will have major repercussions on the perception and comprehension of the person's situation and circumstances.

Almost everyone thinks that dementia is simply loss of memory of different degrees. It has been defined as a memory disorder. Memory is obviously very important. We need to be able to *make and use* new memories until the day we die, but there is much more to dementia than just loss of memory.

Memories can be damaged, they can decay, and they can mutate. We only need to examine our own memories realise that this is true. Memories need to be constantly added to, renewed, and restored. Again, think about what continuing professional development does for you. If this replacement and restoration does not occur, the memory stores become depleted and there is less total information and minimal current information available for processing in response to need of a capable cognitive response.

For the purposes of understanding, we divide memory into different areas. We should recognise that these divisions are academic models and do not necessarily reflect what happens in real life.

First, we divided into *short-term* and *long-term*. A lot of people believe that the loss of short-term memory is not serious, 'it's only her short-term memory'. However, short-term memory, what happens in the brain in the immediate and short term, has important functions, of which remembering something that was said recently is only one.

We are continually immersed in information. Look around, listen, smell. We handle a lot of information that is only temporarily relevant or not obviously relevant at all.

Its most important function is *working memory*. In the psychological literature there is debate whether working memory is part of or separate from 'short-term memory'. In my handout, I use the heading 'short-term memory and learning', as the things that happen at the beginning of memory cycle.

Working memory is what enables learning. I believe that learning starts with the intent to learn. That intent depends on perceived relevance. As I have mentioned previously, in any situation we are surrounded by sensory information that we make no effort to commit to memory. Something, and I believe it to be *executive function*, triggers the intent, and hence the effort to learn.

Think back, how many of your patients have questioned the relevance of items in the MMSE and the MOCA? 'This is nonsense ... I haven't done anything like this since primary school.' How many angry relatives have you heard complain that dad lost his driver's licence because he couldn't spell 'world' backwards.

For example, we may look up a phone number, dial it and make a call. We may have no further use for that number, and there is no point in memorising it, and it decays after a few moments.

If the phone number was one that I was likely to use again and again, I would make the effort to learn it. As a student, I learned a lot of information for a purpose such as an exam that I made no effort to retain in the long-term. In the middle of the medical course, I enrolled for Psychology 1 for interest. It turned out not to be what I expected, so I stopped attending. In those days, no one kept careful watch on what the students were doing. I decided to sit for the exam, so the night before, I read right through the textbook. I passed the exam, and promptly forgot the subject. Had it been important and relevant, I would have made efforts to maintain these memories, and would probably still be able to access them to this day.

To learn something, we must be capable of concentration on several types of selected information simultaneously in an orderly and purposeful manner. We must *create a package that consists of the core of information and relevant associations.* In the psychological literature they are called chunks. To do that, we must focus on it long enough to enable the brain to capture it, consolidate sufficiently so that it will be captured, consolidated more completely, and stored in long-term memory. Thus, we cannot have long-term memories without short-term memories. In computer terms, this is like RAM. We decide what information we are going to want in the future and save it in the database on the hard disk. That information will then be available the next time we boot up and can be retrieved any time that we need it.

When we do cognitive testing, we give the person a learning task (learn three words in the MMSE, five words in the MOCA) to complete, and then ask them to repeat these words, immediately in the case of the MMSE, and after a delay with distractions in the MOCA. The registration task is scored in the MMSE (three points), which I consider to be a freebie. Only complete recall is scored in the MOCA test, but the response to category and multiple-choice cues is also tested. Many people, who scored zero on recall, will respond to some of the prompts. The way that I view this is that the core information has not been retained, but some of the associations have. We all use associations in our recollections and the inability to do so is a significant loss.

For similar academic reasons, we divide long-term memory into specific areas. The first question that arises is when does short-term become long-term? The answer is, when the new memory becomes fully consolidated.

What's in a word? A great deal. *'Long-term memory' has become synonymous with 'old memory'.* As I explain below, all of our mental processes are fuelled by memory. To be useful in dealing with our lives, the information that fuels the mental processes must be current. Our semantic, episodic, procedural, and yet unnamed memories must be current. They must be new and not old.

What we call *semantic memory* is memory for knowledge, facts, things we have learned. In the interview and from the testing it becomes obvious that the patient remembered less information than she would have been able to in the past. This is not entirely about recall, as memories decay and probably 'use it or lose it' applies. I believe that semantic memory is most subject to decay, because it is the least likely to be replaced and consolidated unless it remains completely relevant. With cognitive impairment, we are also not adding new information to the long-term stores, which therefore become depleted.

What we call *episodic memory* is the memory of things that have happened to us, events, our autobiography. This is what most people think of when they talk about long-term memory. Often, we believe that anything that somebody tells us in detail from the distant past must mean that they have a good memory, but we have no way of verifying this most of the time. During my assessment, I have two ways of testing episodic memory. The first is by taking the medical history. Relatives are often quite surprised that mother, who remembered what happened at Auntie Mabel's wedding in 1948 in enormous detail, did not recall that she had had a coronary bypass, a fractured femur or a hip replacement. The other way is to take a biographical history, which we should all do if only to determine the educational level that can dictate our choice of screening tests and their interpretation.

I believe that episodic memory is more robust than semantic memory but less then procedural memory. We celebrate happy events, such as birthdays and wedding and thereby we consolidate the memory. We commemorate the deaths of loved ones as well as their achievements. We remember horrendous events because they haunt us as in PTSD.

There is third type of long-term memory called *procedural memory*, that most people don't understand is a form of memory. This is the memory of all the complicated things we learn to do throughout our life, like tying shoelaces, riding a bike, driving a car, baking a cake or playing the violin. We don't think of them as memory because we don't access them in the same way as semantic and episodic memories. To recall facts or events we must make a conscious effort to remember.

The procedural memories are all complicated series of actions that must happen exactly in a very orderly, identical sequence every time. You don't get in your car, turn on the ignition, and then try to remember what you are supposed to do next. You drive off, you may arrive safely at a destination with no exact memory of how you did it. The information retrieval is happening at such a rapid rate that we are not conscious of it. It is subconscious and it is continuous, adjusting to a changing context and environment. Even though it does not behave like semantic and episodic memory, like them it is memory that can be damaged and lost.

Rigid separation into forms of memory is not what happens in real life and does not explain what actually happens. I demonstrate this by explaining to a partner or a relative how a simple action such as picking up a pen and then talking about it involves all aspects of memory. I have a purpose in mind, and a short time was spent in working memory. I have semantic memories of it. I know what it is, I know what it does, I have used it in a specific way several times, and quite recently. I have episodic memories of it. I picked it up without thinking, I triggered a procedural memory. There is lots more however, I can see it and touch it, the sensory system is involved. I am waving it around; the motor system is involved. Thus, in this simple action not only every type of memory, but other parts and systems of the brain have been involved, and my purpose of picking the pen up to explain what was happening in the brain was achieved. Procedural memories are the most robust because of the constant repetition.

This brings us to the next topic. Something continuous and highly coordinated is happening that reflects our intent and purpose, that monitors our interaction of every kind with our environment, that enables us to reason, plan, organise, access all the information that we need to be aware of our circumstances, and triggers our procedural memories in response to changing circumstances. It is called *executive function*. It is based in the front part of the brain, but it is connected to every other part of the brain to enable all of the above to occur. It can be damaged and ultimately lost in severe or progressive dementia, when its inter-connections are lost.

High level example of procedural memory and executivefunction

Driving is an exceedingly complex multistage procedural memory. We often have little memory of completing a trip when we arrive at our destination. We run on 'automatic'. However, no two trips are the same, and we must have made numerous adaptations to current circumstances subconsciously. It is only when something unexpected happens that we must make rapid conscious decisions and responses. The routine, uncomplicated part of the journey was being monitored and adapted largely subconsciously.

What if a very, very experienced driver driving entirely 'on automatic' is confronted with a completely unexpected crisis, such as another vehicle, a person, an animal emerging very unexpectedly in front of him? Would he have the capacity, based on the depleted memory stores left to him, and the necessary executive function to react quickly and appropriately, given that there are now threats to the safety of persons other than himself?

Basic example of procedural memory and executive function

Mrs Bloggs has severe dementia. It is dinner time and she is very hungry, sitting at the dinner table at her nursing home. A carer places a plate of soup in front of her, and nothing happens... Until the carers says, 'Pick up your spoon dear and eat some soup'. She eats, stops, and must be prompted again. What should have happened was that as soon as the plate of soup was put on the table, she should have picked up her spoon and polished it off. This should have been triggered by EF. In the absence of EF, it needed external prompting, talking her stepwise through the activity.

I have seen many situations where a family has become alarmed by mother's weight loss. They surround her with food. They bring meals, there is food in the fridge, the freezer, the larder, and anywhere else that food can be located. They organise Meals on Wheels. Mother continues to lose weight. The food goes uneaten, and the dog gets fatter. When they bring mother home for a meal or go out together, she eats like a horse. Eventually, it becomes apparent that mother needs to be reminded to eat.

These two examples are at the opposite end of the complexity of procedural memory from driving.

Executive dysfunction, not memory loss as measured by simple cognitive testing, is the most significant impairment in dementia. It must be looked for in every assessment. This does not mean performing the Frontal Assessment Battery but seeking real life evidence from the people that have the closest contact with the patient.

Delusions are false beliefs that are commonly found in dementia. The criteria that define delusions are:

- certainty (held with absolute conviction),
- incorrigibility (not changeable by compelling counterargument or proof to the contrary),
- impossibility or falsity of content (implausible, bizarre, or patently untrue).

There are several theories about the causation of delusions. In the context of dementia, I believe that they are disorders of perception of the situation, information processing, and distorted reasoning that is based on these misperceptions.

They are common, and if looked for can be found quite 'early' in dementia (when there is a high MMSE score). They may be frightening and distressing for the person. They can cause great stress on the relationship. 'He makes things up ... He tells lies about me ... He's become very argumentative.' When I had asked the patients about whom such comments had been made, about their concerns, they had responded with, 'It's my wife. She is trying to run my life, always arguing, always telling me what to do.'

Fully blown, they can make life with the patient unbearable for the partner. Partners and families argue about the accusations made about them, such as stealing. 'He won't abide having our son-in-law, Rod in the house. He says Rod stole his tools, but I was there when he gave them to him.'

The relief when delusional thinking is explained is palpable.

Hallucinations, alone or combined with delusions can also make life very difficult. The man who believed that there was someone else living with them every time he went past a mirror, insisted that his wife set a place at the dinner table for that person, and it was easier to comply than argue with him.

Some form and degree of anxiety is virtually universal in dementia.

Anxiety is a persistent sense of fear, disquiet, & uncomfortable restlessness. Common presentations include *general anxiety*, where virtually everything makes them anxious and they are continuously on the edge.

Anticipatory anxiety is also common. I have often been told that the patient had been worried about our upcoming appointment ever since they learnt of it, and that they did not sleep the night before, and tried to cancel the appointment right up to the last minute.

Social anxiety is supposed to happen to adolescents, who avoid new social situations for fear that they will not cope and will appear to be 'uncool', nerdy, or gawky, to their peers. This can often occur the other end of the age spectrum.

Separation anxiety, which is the fear that babies and tots have if separated from their mother, is quite common and distressing in dementia, often quite early in the presentation. It is the morbid fear that the most important person, usually the life partner, is going to abandon, or has already abandoned the patient. It reaches delusional proportions.

It is enlightening to look at the DSM-V diagnostic criteria for separation anxiety, including adult separation anxiety:

- Recurrent excessive distress when anticipating or experiencing separation from home or from major attachment figures.

- Persistent and excessive worry about losing major attachment figures or about possible harm to them, such as illness, injury, disasters, or death.

- Persistent and excessive worry about experiencing an untoward event (e.g., getting lost, being kidnapped, having an accident, becoming ill) that causes separation from a major attachment figure.

- Persistent reluctance or refusal to go out, away from home, to school, to work, or elsewhere because of fear of separation.

- Persistent and excessive fear of or reluctance about being alone or without major attachment figures at home or in other settings.

- Persistent reluctance or refusal to sleep away from home or to go to sleep without being near a major attachment figure.

- Repeated nightmares involving the theme of separation.

- Repeated complaints of physical symptoms (e.g., headaches, stomach-aches, nausea, vomiting) when separation from major attachment figures occurs or is anticipated.

Practically every item can be found when structured histories are obtained from the patient and the partner.

In both delusional states and anxiety there may be a very high level of arousal which results in a high state of vigilance and a fight or flight response that can make it very difficult to engage the person and use nonpharmacological methods of dealing with their disturbance.

Depression, often inseparable from anxiety is also common. There may be a sense of hopelessness that leads to withdrawal from normal participation in social activity and a wish to end life passively or actively. This is the ultimate distress.

I am very attracted to the principles that underlie Cognitive Behaviour Therapy. The most attractive feature is that it focuses on the problem, the manifestation, rather than the speculated causes like its predecessor, psychoanalysis. It is practical and immediately applicable.

I believe that in dementia, because there is a failure to form new memories and thus to update and replenish the long-term memory stores. I also believe that executive function controls and coordinates all mental processes including perception, comprehension, and reasoning. All mental processes are fuelled by information. When that information is out of date and damaged, and when executive function itself becomes impaired, the afflicted person interprets situations with the only information available to her and reacts accordingly.

The cognitive distortions outlined by Aaron Beck and David Burns again resonate with my beliefs and observations.

- Always being right
- Blaming
- Disqualifying the positive
- Fallacy of change
- Fallacy of fairness
- Filtering
- Jumping to conclusions
- Labelling and mislabelling
- Magnification and minimization
- Overgeneralization
- Personalization
- Should statements
- Splitting (all-or-nothing thinking, dichotomous reasoning)

Studying each of these in detail again resonates with what I find in a detailed clinical case taking.

It is relevant to understanding the thought processes of people with delusional thinking and anxiety. This in turn gives us targets that can be addressed in behavioural interventions of all kinds.

Progression of dementia

The progression of dementia is most easily understood by recourse to a diagram. The upper horizontal line labelled *Cognitive Capacity* is set at the point where all of the cognitive functions (memory, executive function, thinking etc.) are at their peak (normal for that individual).

The lower line labelled *Cognitive Decompensation* (the point at which all cognitive functions are severely impaired and behavioural issues emerge) is the point at which community living becomes impossible.

The diagonal line is the *trajectory of the disease*, which is basically progressively downwards.

The area under the diagonal line and above the second horizontal line is what I arbitrarily describe as *Compensatory Capacity* (reserve capacity, the capacity to rebound).

When one sees a new patient for the first time the capacity is always considerably less than 100%, but as noted above, this is not the onset of the disease.

The brain's equilibrium can the disturbed by numerous events described as *stressors* and presents as *delirium*. These include direct damage to the brain, systemic illness, organ failure, injury, surgery, pain, et cetera. If the cause is found and effectively treated the patient is below the lower line temporarily and returns to the baseline on the diagonal line. A severe stressor generally means that the patient is below the line for much longer and does not return to the baseline. The trajectory is altered and the dysfunctional endpoint is reached earlier than would have been the case if the stressor had not occurred. *The lower the patient is on the diagonal line the more vulnerable the patient becomes to what would have been minor stressors only earlier in the past.*

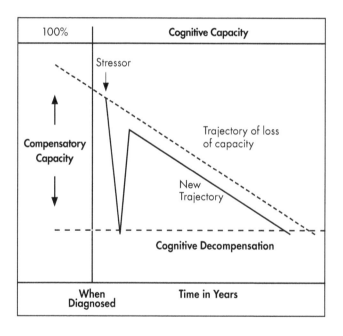

Fitness to drive

Fitness to drive is a very contentious issue and when I have concluded that someone is unfit to drive I go through this document with the partner or relatives and explain how what learned I from the assessment led to that conclusion. I give them a copy to inform other members of the family.

The Ausroads Publication 'Assessing Fitness to Drive' is a valuable and authoritative resource. It describes the driving task very clearly: 'The driving task involves a complex and rapidly repeating cycle that requires a level of skill and the ability to interact with both the vehicle and the external environment at the same time. Information about the road environment is obtained via the visual and auditory senses. The information is operated on by many cognitive processes including short-and long-term memory and judgement, which leads to decisions being made about driving. Decisions are put into effect via the musculoskeletal system, which acts on the steering, gears and brakes to alter the vehicle in relation to the road.'

This repeating sequence depends on:

- vision
- visuospatial perception
- hearing
- attention and concentration

- memory
- insight
- judgement
- reaction time
- sensation
- muscle power
- coordination.

The question that must be answered is: *In a crisis, would this person be able to recognise the risk in the situation and the probable consequences if the action continued without change, be capable of making an appropriate judgement about a response, and then be capable of putting that response rapidly into effect?*

6

Care and Management

Supporting living and dying with dementia

What is aged care? In Australia, all aged care has become identified and managed as part of the welfare system and separated and isolated from the healthcare system. It is primarily about accommodation, and providers may make huge profits. Unfortunately, some non-government organisations, and a growing number of private entrepreneurs, also accommodate the sickest and most disabled people in our community. A very high proportion of residents in High Level Care facilities have dementia and, whether it is recognised or not, need palliative care. These residents have complex health-related needs and are very vulnerable to exacerbations of chronic illness and acute health problems that must be met by admission to public hospitals. The facilities are not appropriately staffed, nor do they have the necessary resources to adequately meet the health care needs of their residents.

I contend that where someone is receiving long-term care that is conditional on an assessment (an ACAT assessment) that identifies impairments and disabilities, it becomes a health issue and a responsibility of the healthcare system, and hence the Minister for health. This is so whether that person is in the community or in residential facility. Any facility that deals with residents with continuing and recurring illnesses and severe disability should have the capability to do this properly, with the necessary staff and resources. Long-term care is about much more than accommodation. Lines of clinical responsibility and duty of care should be clearly defined.

Moving residents from facilities to hospitals is traumatic, stressful, and hazardous for that resident, and extremely expensive for the taxpayer. It increases demand and puts pressure on hospitals, affecting the whole system. High-level care facilities should have an Infirmary capacity, where more intensive treatment can be provided under the continuing care of the general practitioner, with access to consultant opinion.

When I think about the purposes of care, I am reminded of Maslow's pyramid of human needs.

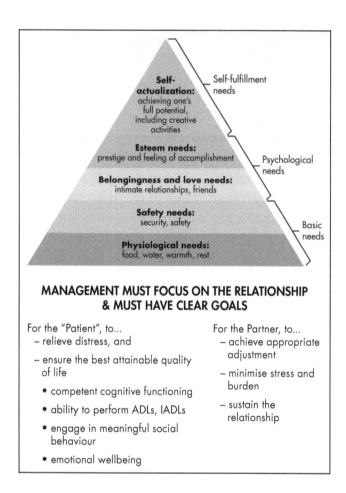

MANAGEMENT MUST FOCUS ON THE RELATIONSHIP & MUST HAVE CLEAR GOALS

For the "Patient", to...
- relieve distress, and
- ensure the best attainable quality of life
  - competent cognitive functioning
  - ability to perform ADLs, IADLs
  - engage in meaningful social behaviour
  - emotional wellbeing

For the Partner, to...
- achieve appropriate adjustment
- minimise stress and burden
- sustain the relationship

Just like everything else about dementia, or any other serious chronic illness, management should be addressed from the bio/psycho/social perspective. The goal of comprehensive care and management is to meet all the needs of people in the context of their current circumstances. In essence, it is to assist people to remain as high as possible on the pyramid. Care and management are the means of regaining and retaining the capabilities of the person and the life partner so that they may function amicably, safely and securely at the highest attainable level.

As health professionals, we have a role to play at every level, but as dementia advances we must operate in the basic needs areas, as these needs cannot be met without good physical and mental health. Without a sound base, the pyramid will collapse.

Home care and residential care are not alternatives, they are different levels of care. The level of care that is most appropriate is the one that meets the needs of the person and the life partner most effectively.

Those who advocate that people should be 'allowed' to stay at home at all costs because they have the right to autonomy often fail to understand that a right to autonomy can only be claimed by people who are capable of acting autonomously; that is who have decision-making capacity. While the law holds that a person has that capacity until proved otherwise, circumstances should be considered broadly. In today's individualistic, person-centred environment, the impact on the life partner and caring relatives, who may not necessarily be living at the same address, is too often overlooked.

Who should be the medical manager?

As I have argued, the Consultant Geriatrician is the most appropriate super-generalist to perform the initial assessment and develop a management plan. To date, we have seen ourselves as super-general physicians, with several special interests, one being dementia.

The whole of general medicine is much too wide a field for geriatric medicine to encompass. People in the age-group that we serve generally have several chronic illnesses, of which dementia is the epitome. The people in this group also do most of the dying in our community, and dementia is now the second most common cause of death. (The top four leading causes of death in Australia in 2015 [ABS]: Ischaemic Heart Disease, Dementia, Stroke, and Lung Cancer. Collectively, these account annually for about one third of deaths.)

To return to some personal history. I was converted to Geriatric Medicine in the early 1970s; while working and studying in England, I had the opportunity to meet, listen to and learn from some of the leaders in British Geriatric Medicine and Psychogeriatrics.

I did not meet Dr Marjory Warren, 'the mother of British Geriatric Medicine'. Well before my time, she had been given the responsibility for the population of a Poor Law workhouse associated with the West Middlesex Hospital in London. She demonstrated that a completely neglected and invisible group of older people could flourish when properly assessed and rehabilitated.

The founders of British Geriatric Medicine applied her principles to a much larger underserved segment of the population, the elderly, people over 65 years old. In modern terms, they moved from the classical medical model to the bio/psycho/social model, and the recognition that the consequences of illness as comprising of impairment, disability, and handicap, all of which are present at any given time, had to be addressed. Marjory Warren was a great pioneer of rehabilitation, which she demonstrated was applicable even to lost causes. For some time, geriatricians became the main providers of rehabilitation to the general population.

Professor Bernard Isaacs gave Geriatric medicine a core focus with his 'Giants of Geriatrics', his four *I*'s: Instability, Immobility, Intellectual Impairment, and Incontinence.

The principles listed above were not being applied in general medicine of the day, and there was little focus on the Giants in any age group. 'The day' was over half a century ago.

Geriatric medicine is now an age-based super-specialty dedicated to the elderly, just as paediatric medicine is dedicated to the young. This made sense when I returned to Australia in the 1970s. Essentially, what we as geriatricians stood for was basically good medicine that should have been applied to any age group. Paediatric medicine is different. It will always be relevant as a super specialty. 'The elderly' is an elusive population subgroup to define with any confidence. It is in no way homogeneous. Wherever we put the boundary, 65+, 75+ et cetera there will be people who are extremely healthy ranging to people who are extremely ill and disabled, and indistinguishable from the rest of the adult population. They should have full and equal access to adult medicine and all its specialties. That is why we need to re-define our niche.

To return to the question, 'Who should be the Medical Manager?' The answer is: *The General Practitioner, assisted on an ongoing basis by The Geriatrician*.

Basic principles of management

Management must focus on the relationship, not merely on 'the patient'; it must be tailored to the exact context; and must have clear goals.

On the completion of a comprehensive assessment, the consultant/practitioner must have a thorough understanding of the issues creating stress and difficulty for the individuals in the relationship. He must also understand the impact that the manifestations have on each of the partners and identify the precise problems that will need to be addressed. He must ascertain the capacity of each to maintain the functioning of the relationship. The non-afflicted partner will have to learn and become capable of playing a new role. The partner is both a recipient and a provider of care.

This understanding cannot be achieved through anything other than a face-to-face, one-on-one consultation with each of the partners. A consultant whose entire experience is shaped by participation in a Multidisciplinary Memory Clinic is not equipped to operate in real life settings.

Management must be congruent with the *context*. By this I mean:

The health context:

- The severity and stage of the dementia
    - Continuing
    - Palliative
    - The Comorbidities and how they impinge on the total care needs, and complicate the management of the dementia

The social context:
- The capacity of the partner

- Physical
- Emotional
- Availability of family support
- Availability of external support, formal and informal

The environment:

- Home/Community
- Supported Accommodation
- Residential Facility
- Hospital

The first step in management is always, Explanation, Education, and Counselling.

Indeed, this is our most important contribution and worth much more than anything that we may prescribe.

Everyone involved in the care of the care of a person suffering from dementia must understand what is happening to that person and their partner, and what their partner's contribution is to the care and support of both, in every setting.

I work primarily in rural and remote communities. The people that I deal with are discriminated against in several ways: they live in rural and remote communities; they are old; and they have dementia and other mental health problems.

However, they have something precious. What they have, that very few people have in modern cities, is a sense of belonging to a caring community. In a country centre, the general practice provides cradle to the grave care. If you are sick or injured your GP will deal with it. If you are admitted to the local hospital, the same GP will be looking after you. If you are admitted into residential care, it will still be the same GP, who will treat you in exactly the same way as in in any other setting. The GP is the conductor of the care orchestra. He has an intimate knowledge of the person, the family, and the community in which they live. He is the only one who has a complete knowledge and understanding of a person's health status, and all the contacts with any element of the healthcare and welfare systems.

In a modern city, you will increasingly have access to a general practice all housed in a spectacular purpose-built surgery, that will guarantee you're seeing a GP in good time at every visit. Unfortunately, you may never see in the same GP ever again. When you are admitted to a metropolitan hospital, your GP will not be taking any active part in your care. When you are admitted into a residential facility, it will be nowhere near where you have been living, and your new GP will be a complete stranger, when you need him most. Ideally, general practices in the city should serve the people in a defined area, akin to a parish, or like a country town. Medicine is not an industry, it is a human service.

Anyone purporting to provide a Consultant Geriatric or Psychogeriatric Service in the rural community must see people face-to-face in that community and learn to understand its strengths and weaknesses. Information gathered by local intermediaries or via tele-consultation is much less then you need to know.

Without this knowledge, we can only make generic one-size-fits-all decisions about management, even though we may be following guidelines and advocating best practice. Which only goes to prove that what we confidently describe as Quality Assurance is nothing of the sort.

Substitute decision-makers

When someone does not have the capacity to make rational decisions by virtue of mental incapacity, someone else has to make decisions on that person's behalf. Traditionally that has been the next of kin.

We now have legally binding Advanced Care Directives where we can appoint someone to be our Guardian, Advocate, Attorney etc. when we are at the peak of our powers and able to make these important decisions.

When such powers are activated, *the Guardian becomes the patient* in respect of legal and ethical obligation.

The Management Plan should reflect addressing the impairment, disability and handicap that are consequences of illness simultaneously. I also believe that there is no situation, or almost any stage of the disease, where *prevention* and *rehabilitation* do not have a role. We should have a permanent prevention and rehabilitation mindset.

Pharmacological and non-pharmacological interventions are not alternatives

All modern guidelines piously pronounce that non-pharmacological interventions should be tried and implemented before we reach for the prescription pad. These guidelines rarely enlarge on such interventions in any detail. We are not talking about alternatives. The way that we deal and interact with patients and residents, their partners and their formal and informal carers, and the therapeutic relationships that we form, is non-pharmacological, but critically important in every situation. There are many non-pharmacological interventions described and available. Some are completely ridiculous, but what they have in common, and what makes them effective, is that some well-intentioned person gives the sufferer their complete and undivided attention in a friendly and sympathetic manner.

Pharmacotherapy in dementia

There are a number of reasons and objectives for prescribing medication in dementia:

- Modifying the course of the dementia
- Dealing with psychiatric and behavioural problems
- Treating co-morbidities, old and new
- Continuing preventive therapies

Modifying the course of the dementia

The available options are very limited and have not changed for a considerable time.

- Cholinesterase inhibitors
- Memantine

I use and recommend them for mild to moderate Alzheimer's disease unless there are any contra-indications. I have some faith in their efficacy but am also influenced by the need for something that patients, partners and relatives recognise as being some form of active treatment, that something tangible is being done.

Dealing with psychiatric and behavioural problems

BEHAVIOURAL & PSYCHOLOGICAL SYMPTOMS OF DEMENTIA
NOT JUST COMPLICATIONS, BUT MANIFESTATIONS
OBSERVED & EXPERIENCED BY THE PARTNER

Symptoms assessed at Patient & *Partner* interviews	Signs assessed by Behavioural Observation by Partner/Carers
• Anxiety	• Agression
• Depressed Mood	• Screaming
• Delusions	• Restlessness
• Hallucinations	• Wandering
	• Culturally inappropriate
	• Sexual disinhibition
	• Hoarding
	• Cursing
	• Shadowing

These are generally considered as complications; however, they are common, and some are detectable from early in the diagnosis when the assessment is properly carried out.

This is the area that gives rise to the greatest controversy, criticism, and complaint about management in residential facilities. It is very easy to stir up frenzied indignation in the media. Much of it is justified, but much is not. It is easy to fixate on scapegoats, but the causes of the problems are systemic, as I have pointed out in the criticism of the aged care system. As expert professionals and members of professional associations we should not only criticise but set an example of good practice.

This is an area where I question the role and value of specialist Psychogeriatric input. In the mental health system that I have to work with, direct access to a psychiatrist has to pass triage by another category of mental health worker. More often than not, this results in a teleconference that does not allow any kind of understanding of the context including family dynamics and other key issues. This results in totally inadequate treatment.

A relatively common problem is Post-Traumatic Stress Disorder (PTSD) appearing late in life. I refer people to the mental health service that I have to deal with in the hope that they will gain access to psychotherapy. Alas, after a teleconference, this rarely happens and the only therapy offered is the prescription of an antidepressant.

PTSD is PTSD irrespective of the age of the person. I believe that any competent general psychiatrist should be able to manage PTSD in any adult and would accept that any serious chronic mental health condition cannot be competently managed by pharmacotherapy alone, but in combination with some form of psychotherapy.

In this day and age, a competent prescriber in any discipline is aware that physiology, pathology and their impact on the pharmacokinetics and pharmacodynamics has to be considered when prescribing for any individual of any age. This does not require enormous knowledge on our parts. Look up the drug in MIMS, and read it carefully, the full PI version. Because I am often dealing with psychopharmacology, one of my library of handbooks is the *Clinical Handbook of Psychotropic Drugs*, by Bezchblinyk-Butler K., et al. (Hogrefe Publishing 2014). It tells me all I need to know about any psychotropic drug and includes useful 'tricks of the trade' that are not found in general references.

What I have said about PTSD applies to any psychiatric diagnosis found in DSM-5 (the latest version of the American Psychiatric Association's Statistical and Diagnostic Manual of Mental Disorders, 'the bible').

The principles of prescribing in long-term care

Because this is the area that causes the greatest suffering and the greatest difficulty in management, I will outline the simple rules for prescribing that I have applied for many years. They are applicable to any condition.

Diagnosis &indications

Diagnosis must be complete and accurate. The specific manifestation to be addressed must be identified and clear treatment goals set.

In every situation, we should undertake a 'risk/harm– benefit' analysis to ensure that the benefits of the course of action that we propose outweigh its disadvantages and risks. *This always depends on the context.*

The hysteria around the use of second-generation antipsychotic agents in residential care, fomented by many of our learned colleagues who added statistics to the outrage, has created a belief that they should never be used. Generic warnings of dire adverse effects are routinely distributed. This is scaremongering.

An agency that deals with disturbed behaviour in residential care, routinely warns people that, 'only 1 in 5 people will gain benefit from an antipsychotic, but 1 in 100 will die, and 2 in 100 will have a CVA [i.e. a stroke]'.

The conditions that cause disturbed behaviour in residential care include delusions and anxiety caused by the inability to comprehend the situation and to perceive threats and malice where there is none. They are distressed and in a high state of arousal. For many, if not most of them, this is the palliative phase of their life. Their behaviour makes it extremely difficult and unsafe for those around them to deliver needed care. In this context (a very common context in residential care), the information about the statistical risks adds unnecessary fear for partners and relatives who feel guilty enough already.

We cannot leave someone in distress, and their basic survival needs must be met. Partners and relatives understand this. I have often been told by alarmed families, who had looked risperidone up in Google and expressed great fear and horror that the GP had prescribed it, 'We didn't understand, nobody told us about mum's behaviour. We wouldn't have complained if we had known.'

The need to understand all the complexities of the context is a powerful reason for personal one-on-one, face-to-face assessment by the specialist personally.

Non-pharmacological alternatives

This is a no-brainer. The way skilled and experienced carers interact with the patient/resident is in itself a non-pharmacological alternative.

The problem with disturbed behaviour is that you must first be able to engage people, and this often needs to be facilitated with medication that lowers arousal and anxiety. This is common in adult psychiatry.

Pharmacology

It is necessary to understand the basic pharmacology of the drugs being used and to select them on the basis of their pharmacological advantages and ADR profiles. This generally means becoming familiar and experienced with a small number of drugs and adopting a somewhat sceptical approach to the introduction of new drugs into one's personal armoury.

As noted above, we should not hesitate to use reference material, and we should be prepared to consult our more experienced colleagues.

The dose

'*Start low, go slow.*' Start with small doses and progress slowly on the basis of frequent monitoring. As an example, the appropriate pace of treatment of hypertension in the elderly has been described as 'a slow seduction.'

Experience has taught me that the above exhortation is incomplete. It should read: 'Start low, go slow ... But get there!'

The regimen

Use the smallest possible number of drugs in the simplest possible regime, in a way that fits into the patient's usual routines.

- Consider if the patient is *capable of self-administration*. If not, ensure that somebody reliable will be 'in charge' of medication administration.

- Ensure that the patient and/or the partner *understands the treatment* and any problems associated with it. Compliance is most effective when the patient has been party to the decision-making process and is taking responsibility for her own care. That is one definition of 'patient-centred care'.

Use drugs on a PRN (*pro re nata*) basis, that is, as the occasion arises, when necessary is problematic in the context of dementia, and particularly in the context of long-term care, we should understand what we are doing when we prescribe in this way. We are asking someone of unknown experience to make a decision to administer a powerful medication, such as an opioid analgesic or an antipsychotic, with scary side-effects and other consequences, on their own initiative. When teaching, I have often asked nurses about how they deal with PRN orders. Not unexpectedly, responses ranged widely from, 'I never give out PRNs' to answers that amounted to 'every time Mrs Bloggs complains, or she won't shut up'. Agency staff tend to be in the 'never' group because they don't know the residents or the patients. The intent of the prescriber should be conveyed to nursing staff and passed on at handovers. Often, PRN medication can be used to prevent pain or disturbance given before an activity or a situation known to affect the patient.

Monitor treatment for efficacy and ADRs

Review the medication at every meeting. Remember my saying, 'The drugs did it until proved otherwise.'

Review

Many drugs prescribed to manage an acute problem become part of the patient's permanent repertoire, even though the indications may no longer apply, and much unnecessary medication may then be consumed for no reason. Importantly the context changes over time.

Medication review should be a routine part of geriatric practice. I see it as my responsibility in every assessment.

Avoid multiple prescribers

Because of multiple prescribers and use of OTC (Over the counter medication, available without prescription) medication, the patient's general practitioner may not be fully aware of all the medications that the patient is using. This information must be properly documented. As a consultant working outside the hospitals, I rarely prescribe for the patients I see, but I make detailed recommendations for medication use that is then prescribed by the GP, who is in the best position to understand everything that is happening to that patient.

Palliative care

The World Health Organization has published numerous reports, guidelines, and authoritative papers on palliative care. The WHO definition that appeals to me is: 'palliative care is the active total care of patients whose disease is not responsive to curative treatment…The goal of palliative care is achievement of the best possible quality of life for patients and their families'.

For a long time, palliative care was seen as the province of oncology, and to this day many of our conventions are based on this perspective. Many patients with cancer have very painful and distressing deaths. They are not the only ones, and it became accepted that people dying of other conditions could have equally difficult and distressing deaths. Such diseases as motor neurone disease, or end-stage organ failure come to mind. They all share a poor prognosis. A lot of definitions of palliative care, which can be very costly, include a time limit, such as three or six months. Cancer, degenerative disorders, and organ failure have a relatively predictable trajectory, and can fit within these financial boundaries.

Many cancer patients and patients dying of degenerative diseases often need the clinical expertise and the full resources of a hospice. Those who do not, and many of those dying of organ failure, can be managed by general practitioners and in less-intensive facilities with consultant support.

End-stage dementia follows an erratic downward trajectory with no clear landmarks. The end-stage may last for several years. Dementia is rarely curable, or even ameliorable, so that is not a landmark. However, when the person is no longer capable of managing even basic activities of daily living independently, unable to communicate their needs effectively, and unable to make even simple decisions affecting their well-being, they are palliative. That describes just about everybody in high-level residential care, where dementia is now the main reason for admission.

It is important to understand this, because this is a critical part of the context within which management decisions are being made. We must now focus on preventing distress of all kinds, physical (particularly pain), emotional, psychological (all of the BPSD's are distressing to the individual), and spiritual.

Chronic non-cancer pain is a very, very important issue at every stage of dementia. I rarely see patients who do not have some form of chronic pain. Opioids are often prescribed and continued in the long-term. They bring with them highly predictable adverse effects. A common one is cognitive impairment that can mimic or exacerbate cognitive impairment from other reasons.

The role of opiates in chronic pain has now been seriously questioned, and we must ensure that we have an up-to-date understanding of how to use them most effectively and safely.

We must ensure safety and comfort and facilitate the attainment of the best quality of life that can be achieved in the circumstances. When all else is lost, the quality of life depends on relationships, particularly the relationship with the life partner, whose own needs must be recognised and addressed.

Everyone involved in that person's care must understand and accept this. I continue to be disappointed that when I have been consulted to deal with behavioural problems in a residential facility, I am the first person who makes it explicit that this is the palliative phase of this person's life.

Summation

In dealing with dementia we aspire to enable the afflicted person and the life partner to continue a mutually satisfying relationship by removing or alleviating the issues that threaten their relationship and by offering support that enhances their quality of life. In the context of advanced dementia the relationship gives a purpose for living and enables equanimity in the face of an increasingly bewildering life.

Management is much more than merely treatment, and Aged Care is much more than supported accommodation.

Ideally, it is long-term or continuing specialised healthcare that begins with diagnosis and continues to the end of life.

Appropriate management can only result from a comprehensive assessment from a bio/psycho/social perspective. Any consultation with a specialist in any situation, be it hospital, clinic, home or an aged care facility, should be done as an Initial Assessment, as described in an earlier chapter.

The specialist should begin with a blank slate, not a preconceived agenda, and follow the same process and protocol as for any other adult patient and to whatever degree is possible. At the very least, the specialist should meet and attempt to engage the patient alone and ideally in that person's in their current environment. For most patients this would be their home or an aged care facility.

Awareness of the context is extremely important. Many of the people seen for the management of behavioural disturbances ('challenging behaviour') both in the community, and particularly in residential facilities, are in the palliative phase of their lives.

Care by people other than partner or family should be based on the formation of a trusting and friendly relationship. It should be seen as an exercise in, or opportunity for, slow-stream rehabilitation and socialisation, and the life partner should be seen as the most important member of the care team.

At the very least, we must be able to offer freedom from distress of all kinds, safety and security, and whatever quality of life is attainable in the circumstances. Ultimately, quality-of-life depends on relationships.

We approach advanced dementia with a sense of me he lives nihilism: there is nothing more that can be done. An aged care facility can only claim that designation if it provides continuing care. It should not just be a house of death.

There is always something more that can be done or that we can do better. Hours spent in front of the TV set contribute nothing to well-being. Every activity should have a purpose.

I believe in the plasticity of the brain. While learning becomes increasingly difficult, some capacity remains. Procedural memories, the hardiest of them all are acquired through repetitive action. Even a small gain can contribute to independent function and self-esteem. This is rehabilitation.

The loss of verbal communication can sometimes be replaced by other modalities such as gesture and sign language.

Everyone we see is deconditioned. Some form of expertly designed exercise performed every day can result in improved mobility, safety, sense of well-being, and quality of life.

About the Author

Dr Ludomyr Mykyta graduated from the University of Adelaide in 1965. He subsequently gained several post-graduate degrees, and specialised in Geriatric Medicine in the UK.

He has had a long career and has held numerous senior appointments in Geriatric Medicine, Rehabilitation Medicine, and Health Administration, around Australia in the Commonwealth and State public services. He has also worked as a WHO Consultant in Aged Care.

With every appointment he remained in active clinical practice.

After his resignation from the Public Service in 2002, as a Consultant in private practice he has focused almost exclusively on the management of dementia in all settings, predominantly in rural and remote South Australia.

He is a Past President of the Australian & NZ Society for Geriatric Medicine and in 2012 he was appointed a Member of the Order of Australia for services to Geriatric Medicine and medical education.

www.ingramcontent.com/pod-product-compliance
Ingram Content Group Australia Pty Ltd
76 Discovery Rd, Dandenong South VIC 3175, AU
AUHW020840300125
406271AU00003B/19